HANDSOME

Based on A True Story of Mental Illness

Written By:
Gary G. McDonald

From Gary G. McDonald

This book is dedicated to the men and women around the world living with mental illnesses. Everyone doesn't know what you're going through on the inside or how you're feeling today, but maybe this book can help people talk about some of the stigmas that surround mental health. I would also like to thank one of the greatest that's ever done radio, Charlamagne Tha God. Through your constant discussions on 103.5 The Beat and spreading mental health awareness throughout your many platforms, people are seeking the help that they need. Angela Yee and DJ Envy, y'all too have displayed tremendous growth, not just on the radio but in business. We thank you. Tameka Mallory and Mysonne we appreciate everything you're doing on the grounds to uplift our people and calling racism for what it really is and what it means to live in two America's. State of Emergency will now be a part of some college curriculums. If you know of anyone dealing with mental health, N.A.M.I is a national organization that can provide assistance.

ISBN: 9798466901894
Gmcdonald480@gmail.com

Gary G. McDonald

Table of Contents

Introduction

Chapter: 1 Leave Him Alone	5
Chapter: 2 My Brother's Keeper	10
Chapter: 3 Beat Them to the Punch	14
Chapter: 4 Growing Pains	16
Chapter: 5 Pick of the Litter	20
Chapter: 6 Gang Related	24
Chapter: 7 N.A.M.I	28
Chapter: 8 Can't get Right	31
Chapter: 9 Suicidal	35
Chapter: 10 Neutralization Through Felonization	39
Chapter: 11 Not My Momma Too	41
Chapter: 12 Inner Demons	45
Chapter: 13 Speed Dating	49
Chapter: 14 Never In, a Million Years	54
Chapter: 15 20 Dwarfs	59
Chapter: 16 What You Not Gone Do	64
Chapter: 17 Naked and Afraid	67
Chapter: 18 Conclusion	78

Acknowledgements

Handsome

Introduction

Donnie's a handsome little boy living in the City of Chicago, born with mental illnesses. Along with the help of his mother and siblings, they all pitch in to try to help him deal with his bi-polar disorder and Schizophrenia. As Donnie gets older, his problems start to pile up and so does his felony convictions. The voices in his head play an important role in how he deals with his issues and life circumstances. Dealing drugs and hanging out on the block was a part of his daily routine. The gang life eventually catches up with him and he's sent to prison. With the deaths of two of his brothers, mother and nephew hanging over his head, Donnie goes into a downward spiral. He later moves to New York to live with his brother, where he's encountered by the Rochester Police, as he walks down the street in the rain naked.

Gary G. McDonald

Chapter 1

Leave Him Alone

It was a cold and windy morning in Chicago and the Prince brothers were ready for the park.

C'mon Donnie, Let's play on this side away from them, John says with a look on his face. I like playing with my friends. You ain't my daddy. You can't make me stop being friends with them. Nan nanny boo boo, John can't catch me, Donnie says jokingly. I'm going to tell mama you're not listening to your big brother. You know she always say listen to your big brother. Right? She's going to be mad at you.

One of the kids from the playground started to tease Donnie. Repeating everything that he would say. John keeps an eye on the kid and tells his brother to ignore him.

Listen to your brother, before your mama beat yo butt, says the kid in the park. You got a problem dirty boy? John asked. Pick on somebody your own size. You don't even know how old I am, said the little boy. I don't need to know. All I do know is that I'm gone beat your lil dirty ass about my brother. Why you got to fight his battles for? Cause I can. He's my brother. That's what brothers are for dirty boy.

Donnie continued playing with his G.I Joe toy action figures. He wasn't paying any attention to what was going on around him. Donnie suffered from bi-polar disorder and schizophrenia. In the 70's his parents didn't have the means of getting him properly diagnosed or in for treatment.

I ain't scared of you neither. My big brother could fight you, and I'll fight him, says the little boy. He could barely speak. Why do you want to fight him? Cause I can stupid. Plus, he act like something wrong with him. Look at how he staring at the tree. Your brother retarded huh? I'm not. Pick on me, John said loudly as he pushes the boy. He won't fight you back, but I will.

The little boy picks up a stick to hit Donnie. John reaches over and grabs the stick from the kid inches before hitting his brother.

Come here with your lil dirty ass, John said after breaking the stick across his knee. I'm gone beat you like you stole something.

Handsome

The little boy runs away from the park to get his older brother. In Chicago, when someone tells you that they're coming back, they mean it. John wasn't sticking around to find out if the boy was bluffing or not, and orders Donnie to get his things so they can leave. Donnie gets his things from the grass and holds his brother's hand.

C'mon Donnie, walk faster. We got to go before they come back with more of his friends or brother. I'm not sure how big his brother is, but these grown ups don't play around. They shoot kids too Donnie. They going to shoot me, John? Donnie asked. Not if I could help it. Ain't nobody messing with my little brother. I will protect you until the day I die. C'mon, speed up Donnie.

As the two brothers hurried along avoiding trouble, John heard someone say, "there they go".

John clutches his brother's hand and started to run. The group of seven boys chased them for several blocks until Donnie stopped to pick up a toy he had dropped. John yanks his arm in frustration and tries to get him to hurry along.

Dang Donnie. Forget about those toys. C'mon, catch up. You're going to get us caught.

A few of the boys cut through a neighbors yard and hop the fence to corner the brothers off in an alley. John thought for sure that they were home free, when suddenly the boys reappear. This time they were armed with sticks, bats and bicycle chains. Leave him alone, we ain't did nothing to yall. He won't hurt a fly. That little dirty boy started all of this. Can yall just let me and my brother go? We don't want any trouble, said John. We finna kick yall ass, someone shouted in a squeaky voice.

John punched the biggest boy there and laid him out cold. The other boys saw blood pouring from his nose and mouth and got scared. They all dropped their weapons and ran in another direction after hearing their friend snoring. None of them wanted to share that same fate.

I told you that I would protect you at all cost. Eventually you're going to have to fight your own battles. I can't always be around, especially at school. I understand John. I'm tough too. I ain't no wimp, said Donnie. I ain't scared of them. I know you're not little brother. As you get older Donnie, you're going to notice that you think differently from other people. We live in the same house, so I get to see your behavior. Other people don't live with us, and some of the things you do might scare them. They might not know how to deal with it like your family can. You understand Donnie? Yea I get it. I think.

Gary G. McDonald

Are boys going to try to fight us all the time because of me John? We not big yet. We're still kids. I'm just telling you to watch out for it. People are going to call you names and say a lot of other mean stuff to you, but you got to stay cool. You have to choose your battles wisely Donnie. Why they going to be mean to me Donnie? Did I do something wrong to all of them? Why people always going to pick n me John? Am I a bad person? You're a good person Donnie and a wonderful brother. Don't let it get to you. I'm wonderful John? You sure are little brother. They lucky Tommy and Bryan wasn't here. They would've been so scared. We would've been like the Chicago Bulls out here.

John and Donnie finally arrives at home and their mother immediately goes off on them.

Where the heel yall been? I asked yall little black asses to beat me here and it's the other way around. I'm a single mother trying to raise 5 kids by myself. This shit ain't easy you know. I'm here to protect you all from the evils that plague the earth. We're sorry ma. Some boys was picking on Donnie and I had to fight them off. You're supposed to help your brother. But I don't give a shit if the sun don't shine, your ass better beat me home from here on out. Understand me? That goes for all of yall, shouts Mrs. Prince. Yes, ma'am everyone says simultaneously. Where is Bryan, Tommy and Shante? I don't know ma. It was just me and Donnie at the park. We're back here Ma, a voice shouts from the backyard. Shante at her friend Hope house across the street. Me and Bryan back here fixing on this bicycle. Go get your sister John. The hell you mean she across the street. I don't know Hope's parents like that to be having my child over there.

Mrs. Prince was very strict when it came to disciplining her kids. Chicago was a very rough city, and many of the boys and girls from those areas didn't live to be teenagers. Although their mother showed them tough love, her kids knew that she had their best interest at heart. Most kids from the neighborhood got to stay outside until the streetlights came on. Not Mrs. Prince kids. They had eaten dinner, did their homework and had a bath by that time. She had a strong hold over their lives and refused for any of them to be a statistic.

Yes ma'am? You wanted me Ma? Shante asked. Who told you that it was ok for you to be going inside of people's house? I know I sure as shit didn't. Get yo ass in there and clean up that bathroom. Yes ma'am. Sorry Ma. I told Bryan and Tommy to tell you. I'll ask next time. It won't happen again. Girl I don't care if you was at church. Get my permission first. Ok young lady? Yall little fast ass girls these days. You better not bring no babies up in here Shante. Both of yall ass gone be in the streets.

Handsome

Yall go bathe up and get ready for supper. Donnie you and John first. Coming in here all sweaty, smelling, and dirty. Wash the color off your ass. I should put a dab of bleach in there to make sure you thoroughly clean. And wash behind your ears boy. Bryan go to the store and get us some Jungle Punch. Ok Ma.

Bryan runs along and Donnie comes into the kitchen with his arms folded.

Boy, what do you want? I don't want to take a bath mama. If you don't get your little ass in that tub and bathe, I know something. I don't want to bathe. I don't feel like it.

Donnie knocked over a cup that was sitting on the counter. Mrs. Prince said a prayer and then counted to ten slowly. She was aware of his mental issues, and often practiced different exercises on how to deal with him or the situation at hand. Mrs. Prince never had Donnie diagnosed or treated for his illnesses, the family just did the best they could. Being a bus driver has also shown Mrs. Prince how to have patience with her passengers as well as her own children. Especially a child suffering from mental illnesses.

Donnie get your ass in that tub boy, before I rip your damn skin off of your back. I be scared Ma. The ghost be in there talking to me. Boy ain't no damn ghost in this house. Could you come with me? Please Ma. Tell John to get in there with you. Show me where the ghost at so that I could beat both of yall ass for playing with me.

Daniel grabs the sides of his head and starts screaming to the top of his lungs. The Prince siblings was immune to their brothers erratic behavior and outburst and have learned to deal with it over time. Mrs. Prince contacted N.A.M.I, which is the National Alliance on Mental Illness. They were a new organization on the rise that assisted family in getting the proper help for the individual or their loved ones. Mrs. Prince thought about calling the ambulance, but that would've meant having the police come out too. She was a smart, praying woman that decided to opt out of having the police come. Over they years, she's read pamphlets and educated herself on the topic of mental health and began to sought out resources before it destroyed her family. Her kids were the love of her life, and the devil wasn't about to wrap his arms around her baby boy.

Good evening. I'm Mrs. Prince. My son Donnie is having an episode. Can you send someone over to assist me with him? We'll send the A Team over as soon as possible ma'am, hold tight. C'mon Donnie, calm down baby, mama right here. Calm down baby. Mommy loves you. Help is on the way Donnie. God please watch over my baby. Please help him to be a strong black man. Help him to deal with this disease.

Gary G. McDonald

Help him to shake this Lord God. My baby too young to be going through this. Send your angels to surround him with their mighty shields of armor. Our father who art in heaven, hallowed be thy name. Thy kingdom come, thy will be done, on earth on earth as it is in heaven. Give us this day, our daily bread and for give our debts as we forgive our debtors. Lead us not into temptation but deliver us from evil. For thine is the kingdom, the power and glory forever. Amen.

Donnie calms down after his mother's prayer and waits for help to arrive.

Am I going to die Ma? Why do I keep screaming and misbehaving? I be trying to be good Ma, but I can't help it. I try not to scream, but it's stronger than me, Donnie says nervously. I can't stop my hands from shaking Ma. Is this normal? It's ok baby. You're ok. Don't worry about your hands right now. We have some people on the way to help you. They're going to try to make you better. The devil won't have the last word in this house. God is the ruler of this kingdom. Satan has no dominion over you Donnie. We're going to fight him off together. Whenever he tries to tell you to do bad things, get on your knees and pray to the lord. The devil only answers when you entertain him. A clown ain't shit without an audience Donnie. You have to learn to fight him. Those voices in your head is the devil trying to talk to you. Trying to get you to do bad things. Learn to ignore him baby. I hear the A Team pulling up outside. C'mon Donnie. Everything's going to be alright baby. You'll see. Just say your prayers for momma. Yes ma'am. I love you mama. Love you too Donnie. This is Psalms 23 Repeat after me baby. The lord is my shepherd, the lord is my shepherd. I shall not want. I shall not want. He maketh me. He maketh me. To lye down in green pastures. To lye down in green pastures. He leadeth me. He leadeth me. Beside the still waters. Beside the still waters. He restoreth my soul. He restoreth my soul. Ye though I walk. Ye though I walk. In the valley. In the valley. Of shadow of death. Of shadow of death. I fear no evil. I fear no evil. For thou art with me. For thou art with me. Thy rod. Thy rod. And staff comfort me. And staff comfort me. They comfort me. They comfort me. Thou prepare a table before me. Thou prepare a table before me. In the presence. In the presence. Of my enemies. Of my enemies. Amen. Amen. Go with these nice people. They're going to bring you back in a little bit baby. Are they gonna hurt me Ma? They here to take me away for good. I'm gone be good momma. I ain't gonna cause any more trouble.

Handsome

Chapter 2

My Brother's Keeper

Ma, Is Donnie going to be ok? John asked. Yea baby, he's got a rough road ahead of him. That's why it's important that yall stick together, no matter what. If anything, ever happens to me, I want yall to make sure Donnie is taken care of. He won't do well on his own. Somebody has to keep an eye on him. We know he got problems, and so does other people. They ain't all blind to it, they just laugh in secrecy and behind people's back. Kids are mean, and boys like Donnie going to always get bullied and picked on, Tommy said angrily. I'm my brother's keeper. As long as I'm around, nobody's laying a finger on him, said John. Yall get to this dinner table. Ain't nobody fighting nobody. They're going to put your brother on some medications. It's up to all of us to make sure he's taking them regularly. If he misses a dose intentionally or by mistake, you'll notice immediately. He's going to have some good days and bad days. He's family. Let's just continue to pray for him and hope that he grows out of it. Through Christ, all things are possible. Amen. Amen, the kids say simultaneously. The world is cruel and full of evil. The devil's going to be coming at Donnie with everything he's got. That's the guilty party. He's responsible for the breakdown of black families. The robbing, raping, and murders our people commit. They're all acts of the devil. Why you think I keep yall in church? We're fighting a spiritual warfare. There are unforeseen dangers and demons waiting to get their hands on black kids. I pray for yall all day and night. It's only so much that momma can do. The rest is up to you, you and you. I hope each of yall paying attention, because this ain't a game. Just be good kids, watch out for your brother and stay out of trouble. I work my ass off driving buses to provide a good life for you kids. Donnie need all of you. I need all of you to do what's right. Do right by each other. Shante hook him up with one of your friends, Tommy said jokingly. Shut up big head. I can't stand you. Ma look, Tommy making fun of Donnie right after you just told us to help him. She sticks out her tongue as she snitches on him. Ma being serious. Stop making jokes. So immature, Shante says nonchalantly. Just do as I said, Mrs. Prince shouts. Donnie should be released shortly. Make him feel comfortable. Don't be asking no stupid ass questions Bryan and Tommy. Don't ask if people were beating their heads on the wall. Just let him come home and rest. Donnie don't need to be answering any questions right now. He's going through a lot. We all are, said Mrs. Prince. Talk to him like normal. If he bring up that place, try to change the subject. I don't want him dwelling on the past and what's happened today. It's bad enough we're living in a rough city, he don't need to be made fun of in his own home.

Gary G McDonald

I know siblings get into it all the time, but don't use his mental illnesses against him. Ok? Yes ma'am, the kids say in unison. I need each of you to step up and dig deep. Be your brother's keeper. Don't worry Ma, we will, Joe said with authority. Good. Now let's eat. Bow your heads for grace. Lord, bless this food we're about to receive. Bless those that are sick and suffering and have no food on their tables. Bless those that are in positions to help others. Keep your arms wrapped around all of my children. Amen. Amen.

There's a knock at the door. It's the facility dropping Donnie off. He was looked over thoroughly and given some medications for his illnesses as well as phone numbers for counseling resources.

I'll get it. Yall gone ahead and eat, said Mrs. Prince.

She looks through the peep hole and see's Donnie standing there with a counselor and opens the door.

Hey mama baby. I miss you. It's a lot of food on the table, go eat. Hi, I'm Samantha his caseworker. Hi, I'm Donnie's mother, Cynthia. Can we sit and talk for a minute Cynthia? Sure, right over here. Donnie's been diagnosed with bi-polar disorder and schizophrenia. These disorders are serious business. They affect how a person thinks, talks, feels and behave. Donnie needs around the clock monitoring. Ma'am I won't lie to you, it's not going to be easy. He's going to have outburst and other behavior that people will think is weird. A lot of his conversations and thoughts will be out of touch with reality. Donnie will have to undergo lifelong treatment. He will also need to take a substantial amount, of meds to keep balanced. It's an uphill battle ma'am. With a lot of love, support and continuous counseling, he'll be able to stay on track. I'm a praying mother Ms. Samantha. God will get us through this. I've never had anything come to me easy. I had to struggle for everything I have. This won't be no different. I'm determined for my kids to be successful and have a better life than what I had. You paly the hand your dealt. Period. I wish the best for you and your family ma'am. Yall be safe. This is my card. Call me day or night. Let me walk you out. Nice meeting you Mrs. Prince. Same here Samantha. I really appreciate all the help. If you have any questions regarding his meds, treatment or anything, don't hesitate to reach out.

The women shake hands and go their separate ways. Mrs. Prince walks back toward the kitchen and wipe away her tears of sorrow. She's witnessed firsthand one of her cousins deal with multiple personality disorder and depression.

Handsome

Hey kids. Hey Ma. Donnie eating like they ain't feed him in there. See that's the dumb shit I was talking about earlier, said Mrs. Prince. He just walked in and you bumping your gums already. Boy sit yo ass down and worry about yourself. Yes ma'am, Timmy says embarrassingly. I don't care if he ate the whole damn table, he's still your brother. And hurry up and go clean up that damn room. Big head ass.

The other kids snicker under their breaths. Yall over there grinning like a Cheshire cat? No ma'am. Remember what we discussed about my brother's keeper? Alright now. I don't want no shit later. Mrs. Prince reiterated. Clean off the table and wash these dishes. Whose night is it to clean the kitchen? It was Donnie's night, but I'll do it for him, John said enthusiastically. You ain't got to tell me twice, said Shante. I guess that's settled, Timmy mumbled. I'm going to take a bath and lay down. Love yall. Them white folks got the butter from the duck today. My feet hurting so bad. I need to soak them in some Epson Salt, or bathe in some Calgon. I'm moving on fumes. Ain't nothing else left in mam's tank. I gotta recharge my batteries. Get you some rest Ma, we got this, said Shante. Ok baby girl. Keep your brothers in line for me. You know where I keep my belt right? If they get out of line Shante, you got my permission to tear on some asses. Mrs. Prince said jokingly. Ok Ma. Yall heard that. I'm in charge. Anybody get out of line I'm getting the belt. I'm the oldest. How she get to? Never mind, said Tommy.

Shante rolls her eyes at Tommy and smile. John cleans off the table and washes the dishes for his younger brother. Donnie was excited to be back home with his family.

Did yall miss me when I was gone? Of course, we did. It wasn't the same around here without you. We were all worried about you, John said cautiously. Mommy was crying and so was Shante. You can't be scaring us like that Donnie. I'm sorry yall. I didn't mean to. I'm sorry Shante. Sorry John. Sorry Tommy. You believe me right John? Of course, I believe you brother. I know you wouldn't hurt a fly. Yes, I will hurt a fly. Let him get on my food. You'll see what I'll do to him. I seen other people hit flies too, Donnie says with a puzzled look on his face. Don't worry Donnie. It was a figure of speech. You always have my back John. When I get rich one day, I'm gone give you a lot of money for always helping me. You'll see. You damn right. Look out for your brother Donnie. I'm telling mama you cursed. How you going to snitch on the only person that got your back? John asked. I was just playing John. I ain't no snitch. Ok, I'll let you slide this time. We don't snitch on each other. Mama gave me permission to put that belt on yall if you misbehaving. Shante taunts them. Who in here cursing? Shante asked jokingly. Girl, I'll take that belt and use it on your lil nappy headed ass. I'm the oldest. I didn't give a shit what mama told you, John whispered. Ma, John in here cursing, Shante says faintly. So, watch out sucker.
      Gary G. McDonald

If you give me a dollar, you could curse as much as you'd like. Girl I ain't about to pay you so I could curse. I'm your big brother. Stop playing yourself, said John. Get out of here. It's grown men talking. Where at? All I see is two ugly big headed boys. Your voice ain't even deep. You ain't got no hair on your chin. You is a little boy. Clean up this kitchen and be quick about it. I'm in charge. Chop chop. Don't make me come back in here. Girl go to your room and get out of here. Ugly self, Donnie mumbles. I know you ain't talking slow po. Shante says with her arms crossed. Mama would kill me if I said what I really wanted to say. I'll hurt your little feelings. Don't let John boost your head up to get read up and down in here. Shante don't play that. Let me just shut up. Mama said if you don't have anything nice to say, don't say anything at all. Bye yall. Whatever says John. Donnie, we have to teach you how to fight. You can't be scared or running from these kids. They'll always pick on you if you don't fight back. Some of these punches might hurt that you feel from us, but it's only to make you tougher. We're not trying to hurt you. People are always going to test you because you're different. I'm ready to learn how to fight John. I'm tough. I won't cry. I know that you're tough, that's why we're going to show you. We're going to do pushups, sit ups and train you to fight anybody that get's in your face. We'll run this town. Everybody will be scared of the Prince brothers. We'll be the toughest, roughest, meanest brothers on the block, said John. We need a name for our crew. I got it John. The PB's. That sound like trouble don't it John. It does. It's bad ass Donnie. It has to sound worse than that. A little more scarier. What about PB4? Prince brother 4. It's four boys, right? Donnie asked. You're right bro. We gotta ask them what they think about it. I overheard yall talking. It sounds good to me, said Tommy. After a goodnights sleep, we'll get started first thing in the morning.

The Prince brothers got themselves hours of sleep, as Donnie sat up throughout the night staring at the ceiling. He heard noises and voices coming from the closet. The voices was telling him to burn down he house with everyone in it. He tried waking up his favorite brother John, but he was sound asleep. After hours of sitting up frightened, Donnie said his prayers. Hi God, I'm Donnie. I know how to pray a little bit, but I just wanted to talk to you. I don't know how much it will cost to fix me, but I will pay anything. I'm tired of being bullied and picked on God. Do you know why you made me like this? It makes me sad to be like this. Ain't nobody going to want to be around me. Girls ain't gonna like me. I just want to be like other kids God. Does it cost a lot to start over and give me another brain? Could you make me smart and tough like John? I would really like that. Besides mama, I feel that he really cares about me. I just want to think like other people. I will pay anything. I don't have much right now, but I can pay you back when I get bigger. My mama don't have the money either. Love you God. See what you can do for me. Amen
        Handsome

Chapter 3

Beat Them to The Punch

The next morning it's 32 degrees in Chicago. The boys are up bright and early, ready to train their brother Donnie.

Donnie you gotta put on your thermals. It's cold as hell out there. John shouted. It ain't cold. I'll go out there with my shirt off, said Donnie. I'll punch the cold in the face and make it freeze. Let me at em. Bryan and Tommy yall ready? I was born ready bro, Tommy replied. We showed you how to fight. What you mean are we ready little brother? Don't forget you're younger than us. C'mon yall Bryan says as he reaches for his black jacket. We got moves to make. Let's bounce.

The brothers go out back to teach Donnie how to defend himself.

Put your hands up like this Donnie. Cover your face. You gotta be looking to your side using your peripheral vision, Bryan said with authority. What's that? It's when you're looking out of the corner of your eye. Keep your guard up and punch with your right hand.

Bryan and Tommy demonstrate as Donnie and John watch.

Now punch with your left hand, while you're still covering your face. I'm going to take a swing at you Donnie. I want you t duck. When you come up, punch with your right hand to my stomach, said Bryan.

Bryan gets in position. Donnie puts up his guard eagerly awaiting his big brother to strike. He had the eye of the tiger. Tunnel vision. Bryan swung at Donnie's head. Donnie ducked as he was told. He came up with a punch to the ribs.

Damn little brother. That was a vicious punch. You seem like a natural. We might be out here for nothing yall. Get back in position Donnie. Put your guard up. You ready Donnie? Yea Bryan.

This time Bryan took two swings to switch things up. Donnie bobbed and weaved and hit him in the groin area.

Fuck bro. Goddamn it Donnie! We're done practicing for the day. Bryan mumbles. I didn't mean to Bryan. I'm sorry. Are you ok? Yea I'm good little brother. You gotta mean jab there. That's your secret weapon when people mess with you. Punch them right where you hit me, as hard as you can. If you do it right, they'll be on the ground like I am, Bryan says jokingly. Somebody get me some milk out the fridge. Please! Bryan shouts.

Gary G. McDonald

No more practice. That's it for the day. Donnie's a natural. Pure Prince blood. We come from a long line of fighters in our family. I'm talking about some of the best that ever did it. Hands of stone, one of our cousins had. They used to call him Rock. We out here worried about Donnie. We need to be worried about the people he come across that threaten or bully him. I have confidence little bro could handle himself. He's cock strong. Always beat your opponent to the punch. What's an opponent Bryan? Your Op, the opposition, enemies, haters. You know. Mama don't want us fighting, but she's not out there. These boys be carrying knives, guns, bats, chains and whatever else they could get their hands on. You can't get caught slipping out here. You gotta always be on your P's and Q's, said Bryan. Them apartments Cabrini Green where they filmed the tv show Good Times, they don't fuck around over there. Sometimes people go in there and never come out. They kill all of us. Make sure yall never set a foot by that place. Promise me. We promise Bryan. Niggas get killed everyday over there. I don't want it to be any of you. I love my family and I don't want us going through that. Mama will go crazy if something happened to us. You're going to be a good fighter one day Donnie. Keep at it little bro. Practice makes perfect. Will I be as good as you Bryan? Donnie asked. Better than me. Way better. You can't go around starting fights because you're good at it Donnie. You gotta have a reason to beat a nigga's ass. If they start with you Donnie, finish it. If you lose and come home crying, we gonna jump you until you come home with a win. You going hurt me Bryan? I don't want to fight you. I love you. I thought you love me too. I do little bro. You don't get it. It's to make you tougher, not just to be doing it. You'll understand later. Just don't come home crying, and don't let me hear in the streets that you loss. And you have nothing to worry about. If they look like they big and bad and run up on you, punch them in their shit bro. Hit them right in the eye. They'll be blind for a second. That'll give you enough time to get in a bunch of licks Donnie. Once you hear them crying, then you could stop. Not until then. Make them cry like a baby Donnie. You hear me? Bryan asked. I hear you Bryan. I won't forget. You want to practice some more Donnie? Tommy asked. Yea sure. Nah I was just playing. I don't want any of you champ. Get you some rest. Save your energy for the real enemies. We won't always be with you Donnie. Your little ass better join a gang or something if shit get crazy. We did. Me and Tommy. They'll have your back for sure. John and Shante closer to you in age, so they'll be watching out for you at school. Ok, Tommy. If I get into a fight, you coming to help me? Donnie asked. If I'm around, I sure will, said Tommy. Do like Bryan said, and you'll be good. Let people talk all they want. If they put their hands on you, kick their asses. Once you make an example out of the toughest boys, everybody else gone be scared to try you. Key word, "beat them to the punch". John yall the closest. You're responsible for him. That's cool with me, I like to fight anyways. I had a little boy snoring yesterday. Ok Muhamad Ali. See yall later, said Bryan.
                                          Handsome

Chapter 4

Growing Pains

Several years have gone by and PB4 have gotten into more fights than they could count. The majority of those fights were because of Donnie's run ins with neighborhood boys teasing him about his mental illness. His erratic behavior made him a constant target. Everywhere they would go, people would always ask what's wrong with your brother. It was always a topic of discussion and was becoming annoying to Bryan and Tommy, who were a few years older. They loved their little handsome brother, but they were getting into fights that was messing up their money on the streets.

Donnie listen, we love you bro. But we've been getting into all kinds of shit, left and right because of you, Bryan said angrily. Did I do something wrong Bryan? You mad at me Tommy? You ain't did nothing wrong Donnie. We're getting older, that's all. We need to hang around people our ages. It's nothing against you personally, we just growing up and going in different directions. Why you picking on him Bryan? John asked. I'm telling him that we're getting older and he has to stand on his own two feet. What happened to what Ma said about being your brothers keeper? John asked. Man, fuck all of that! You roll with him. Yall can be Frick and Frack. Ma just gonna have to be mad. I can't keep doing this. He's your problem now. We're a family. He need all of us. Let him walk in your shadow, said Tommy. I have my own life to live. Somebody gonna get hurt trying to help him. Everywhere we go. What's wrong with your brother? I'm tired of it, Bryan says with an attitude. Tommy ain't you tired of that shit too? Bryan asked. Hell yeah. I nigga rolled up on me the other day about some shit we did to one of his brothers. But the homie pulled out on that nigga and he took off running. If I got beef with someone, it's gonna be because of something I said or did, not something Donnie talking about in his head. Niggas in Chicago have killed for less. I'm over it brother. If we turn our backs on him, ain't no telling what will happen to Donnie, said John. That sounds like a YOU problem. John, you can't honestly sit there and tell me that this shit don't get on your nerves too. It does, I ain't gone lie, but he's still our brother. What if you was slow or had mental problems, you would want somebody to help you too. Well God, didn't have that in the cards for me. My brain is good and intact. I'm about to bounce. Be safe and look both ways when you crossing the streets. You don't want to be my brother anymore Bryan? I'm gone always be your brother Donnie. Nothing can change that. I just want to do my own thing. We'll still see each other at home. Ok. See you later Bryan and Tommy. Do I be embarrassing yall? No Donnie. Don't worry about it bro. I'll see you at home. I love you bro. we need to be around boys our age. Ok? Ok Bryan.

Gary G. McDonald

What you need to be doing is getting one of these little girls to get your dick wet. Bryan says jokingly. Hanging with us won't make that happen. Actually, you'll be cockblocking us. How you know I ain't did it already? Donnie asked. Boy you shooting dog water. Your little ass couldn't bust a grape. Tommy laughed. Like I was saying, find you something else to do. Don't be a tag along. I can handle my own Bryan you watch and see. That's the spirit little brother. Just keep taking your medication Donnie and you'll be fine. I'm not trying to be mean, we just need our own space little bro. When you get older, you'll understand. You just mad I look better than you Bryan. Look at you, then look at me. I'm the winner. I'm the lady's man, not you. They won't be around for long when you start wilding out on them. That's why I said take your meds. You don't want to scare them off little bro. I'm out. Bye big head. Them medications be making me feel like blah. Some days I don't want to get out of bed. You don't know what it's like inside of my head John. I can't help how I was born. I wish I wasn't like this, but I can't do anything about it. This could've easily been Tommy or Bryan with this disease, and they wanna pick at me. Did you know that Albert Einstein, Van Gogh, and millions of other famous people had mental illnesses John? No, I didn't know that. Vincent Van Gogh was a famous painter a hundred years ago that cut off his own ear. I think his girl cheated on her, and it was a gift. Huh? John asked. Are you sure Donnie? That sounds weird. People like us are weird. We're the weirdos. People always laugh at us and judge us cause we crazy. You're not crazy brother. You're just misunderstood. That's all. You're not crazy, said John. When he cut off his ear, do you think his family cut him off too. You think they called him retarded or crazy? I'm almost certain they did. I definitely would've called him crazy, especially over a girl. That was some crazy ass shit. You know how bad that must've hurt? If you cut your own finger by accident or on purpose, it'll hurt. Who does that? So, what are you saying? You cutting off your ear next Donnie? No stupid. I ain't crazy. He was. I'm good. I was just saying that they're famous and have problems like me. Their illnesses didn't stop them from being great. I'm going to be great at something too. Watch and see John. So, you about to be famous Donnie? John asked. Maybe. Who knows. You never know what God has planned. Hopefully you'll be able to get us out of this bad neighborhood into a big mansion. Mama gone have her own room, and we'll be on the other side of the house, it's going to be so big. She'll never see us unless we want her to. You got my back and I have yours forever John. Thanks for always being a good brother to me. You ain't never pick on me or try to beat me up. You're my favorite. You're my favorite too Donnie. Dress warm, it's freezing outside.

The brothers hug and get dressed for school. Although John knew his brother was tough, he still naturally worried about him. Things could go south, really quick.

Handsome

I don't feel like going to school John. The kids are always picking on me. That's why we showed you how to defend yourself. They're just mad because you're smarter and better looking. You took your meds this morning Donnie? Yeah bro, I took them earlier before we left. Alright. We don't need any problems at school. Do your work. If you finish early, don't distract the class. Ask your teacher for more work to do. You're, real smart, so you'll be finish before everyone else. But that's when you get in trouble the most. When you're bored. I promise to be good John and get straight A's. C'mon, we're going to be late.

The brothers headed off to school and crossed their fingers hoping not to bump into any kids from the neighborhood looking for a fight. Unbeknownst to them, that was the last time that they would see Tommy alive. While walking and hanging out with some friends, Tommy was hit by a car that ran the red light. He was killed instantly. His body was thrown over a hundred feet as the driver fled the scene. News of the tragic accident reached his brother Bryan. He immediately starts to cry and goes to find out what happened. Bryan got onto his bike and pedaled as fast as he could trying to get to the scene. By the time he had arrived, the paramedics were already in route to the hospital. Bryan went to the nearest payphone to call his mother with the bad news, that her son was killed by a hit and run driver. He knew that his mother would blame him, since they were the closest. He hesitated momentarily but this was to important to sit on.

Hi good afternoon ma'am. I'm Bryan Prince, my mother is Cynthia Prince. She's a bus driver out on her routes. Could you have her call home, it's an emergency. Thank you, Bryan said nervously. Ok, I'll give her the message. I hope everything's alright young man. Just tell her it's an emergency.

Bryan hopped on his Huffy bike and hauled ass home, waiting for his mother to call. He's never been this nervous and scared in his life. Shante was just getting in from school.

What's wrong Bryan? Tommy dead Tay. What? What you mean dead? Somebody ran the light and killed him. Bryan said as he cried uncontrollably. You sure it was him? Tay asked, as she started to cry.

Tay picks up the phone and call the hospital. A nervous wreck, Tay could barely dial the numbers.

Hi good afternoon ma'am. I heard my brother was hit by a car. Do you have any information? His name is Tommy Prince. Ok. Let me place you on a brief hold while I check on this for you, says the receptionist.

Gary G. McDonald

Tay's heart was pounding through her chest, as she waited for word if it was Tommy or not. Sorry for your loss ma'am, your brother has passed away.

Tay slams the phone down on the receiver and starts screaming. Bryan follows suit. As the siblings wait for their mom to call, in comes Donnie and John from school.

What's wrong with yall? Why you crying Tay? Donnie asked. Tom, Tommy, Tommy dead, Tay says as she stutters. Tommy got hit by a car. He's dead! Tay screams. It's alright Tay. I'm still here. Tommy in heaven with God. Who hit him? Did they catch the person? Do the police know anything? John asked nervously.

Tears began to run down the face of Donnie and John. The house phone rings. John picks it up.

What's so damn important? Donnie Ok? This better be serious. Who is this? This John Ma. Tommy was hit by a car. He's dead Ma. Tommy dead.

Mrs. Prince screamed to the top of her lungs at the school bus terminal.

Not my baby, she sobs. Jesus help me please. Oh God, not my Tommy. I've been a good mother. Why you take my boy? He's a good kid. He don't cause no trouble. Why God? Why? Why God? I take them to church and do everything you ask of me. I pay my tithes lord. Why my baby? Jesus help me. Please! Please Jesus help me. Oh God, I can't take this. Oh God! Why my baby.

The phone hangs up. Mrs. Prince was hysterical at work. Co workers embraced her and tried to calm her down. She screamed as loud as she could trying to get God's attention. Donnie was already dealing with his own mental health issues, now he had the death of his brother on his plate. The voices in his head had gotten louder and wanted him to commit suicide instead of coping with his problems. Donnie continued taking his medication as prescribed and tried to block out the noise. After the burial of Tommy, the house felt even colder. It was quiet place of mourning. There was no laughter or sounds of kids playing. One of Mrs. Prince's heartbeat was gone. Everyone was sad and barely said a word to each other. Their mother stayed in her room all day after taking a leave of absence, staring at old pictures and smelling Tommy's clothes. The boys kept the house clean, while Tay prepared dinner for them. As luck would have it, a stray baby pit bull found his way to the family's doorstep. He recently wondered away from his siblings and found a new home in the midst of their grieving.

                    Handsome

Chapter 5

Pick of the Litter

"Whose dog is that? Donnie asked John." "Where?" "Down there." "I don't know. He looks hungry. He's all by himself. Let's go get him, said Donnie."

The brothers race downstairs to greet their new friend, stomping on the wooden floors.

"Let's name him Tommy." "I don't know about that Donnie. We can't just let a dog in the house. We gotta check with mom and make sure it's ok. He's clean as hell." "Look at his eyes John. They're grey. Let's get him something to eat. He looks to be a few weeks old, said Donnie." We have to get him a dog collar and a chain. We can't leave him outside, it's too cold. I'll train him t be tough like the rest of PB4. He's going to beat up every dog in the neighborhood. I guarantee it. Tommy, you want to watch Martin with me. You ain't got no job Tommy, Donnie says jokingly. You'll like the show. He's funny Tommy. Let's take him in the bathroom and clean him off. He looks clean already John. Well he's not. Ok, C'mon. We're going to take good care of you Tommy. I ain't going to let you get hit by no cars either.

Tommy barks.

Ruff ruff. So, you understand me Tommy? You gotta be quiet. Momma gonna hear you, Donnie whispered. Here, use this towel, John suggest. Throw it away when you're done bro. Momma will kill us if she knew we used her clean towel on a dog. It's not a dog, it's Tommy. She'll understand. Tommy stay still, I'm trying to wash your little dirty butt.

Tommy barks.

Ruff ruff. We could make a lot of money off of him by breeding him with other dogs. We need to find him a dog to mate with asap. We need money to make more money John. I have a vision. Feeding dogs and getting all of their shots and papers ain't cheap Donnie. I know John, but I'm down to try. We can't let Tommy down. We already lost one, we can't lose this one too. I could be a dog trainer. My dogs gonna be tough like me, and like you too John. You think Bryan would loan us some money to buy Tommy some food? Donnie asked. I doubt it bro. We're on our own with this one. He hasn't been himself either. Bryan and Tommy was close like how you and I are. That was his main man. We have to cheer them up John. Maybe the new puppy could put smiles on their faces. What you think? Alright he's clean. Wipe the floor before Ma comes. And get rid of that towel. Throw it out back in a plastic bag.
Gary G. McDonald

Donnie runs into the kitchen and grabs a plastic bag to get rid of the evidence.

Boy, what are you doing? Mrs. Prince asked. Hey Ma. I was throwing out the garbage. Open that bag up. Why is my damn towel wet? What did you waste on the floor? I used it to wash Tommy off. You used it to wash Tommy off? Boy you done lost your rabbit ass mind. I'm sorry. I didn't mean to say that Donnie. It's ok Ma. What the hell you talking about? Your brother in the graveyard. No Ma. I'm talking about this puppy I named Tommy. He just showed up at the door. You got a damn dog in this house boy? I know damn well I ain't gave nobody permission to bring a dog in this house. What kind of dog it is? A Pitbull. Jesus help us, Mrs. Prince shouts. He's not a dog yet, he still a puppy Ma. He won't cause any trouble. He'll be my responsibility, Donnie said happily. That's what worry me. Where he at? He's upstairs with John. Can we keep him Ma? Please. He's going to cheer up the house. He's the new Tommy. You better watch him with eight eyes. If I see any piss or shit on this floor Donnie, it's gonna be you and me. The first ball of doo doo I see, his shitty ass out of here. You hear me Donnie? Yes ma'am. I promise. Thank you, Ma. Love you. Love you too Donnie. You want to see him? He's handsome and smart just like me. I'm gone get him and show you. Don't be running in my damn house. Stay there, ma. Hurry back before I change my mind.

Donnie runs back upstairs to get his new puppy to show him off to his mother. As soon as Donnie walked into the room, he smelled shit.

Eww. This damn dog shitted all over the floor, John said in disgust. Man, he gone get put out. Ma wanted to see him. I thought she was going to be mad at us, but I think by me calling him Tommy put a smile on her face. We dodged a bullet this time. You coming John? Nah, go ahead. I'm gone stay here and clean up and spray some air freshener in here. Ok, thanks John. I owe you one. C'mon Tommy. I'm about to show you to our mama. Behave yourself. Hopefully she likes you. She's been sad since our real brother died. Ruff ruff.

Ma, this is Tommy. Ain't he handsome? Yeah, he is. I like his grey eyes. He looking all pitiful. He could stay for now. Don't make me regret this Donnie. I'm telling you now. This is a huge responsibility. Are you sure you could handle this? I got it Ma. I won't let you down.

Several months go by and Tommy was officially apart of the Prince family. His brown, and cocaine white fur, stood out amongst other dogs. Tommy's body structure was unique, and everyone wanted their dog to fight him. Tommy was beginning to make a name for himself. He had an undefeated record of 11-0. The local gang CVL was taking notice to Donnie and wanted him to join them. He was honored.
                                Handsome

To get into the gang, Donnie had to be initiated. He also had to learn their street codes and handshakes before becoming an official member. His older brother John was totally against it and begged for him to get out. John's pleas fell on deaf ears. Donnie was out on the block selling drugs everyday he came from school. The gang members made him feel like family. He loved his new friends like they were blood brothers and climbed up in rank quickly. Tommy posted on the block with his master, making sure no harm came to him. Donnie was sixteen and making money to feed his dog and family. Things were going good for Donnie until police jumped out on him and his crew. Police found guns, drugs and other weapons on them. Donnie had ten vials of heroin in his pocket and was taken to Juvie. His mother was contacted and told to come pick him up since it was his first offense. Donnie wasn't locked up for no more than two hours and had already gotten into a fight with a rival gang. Mrs. Prince was extremely disappointed in Donnie, so disappointed that she put them hands on him. Like if you were fighting someone on the streets. She tried to contain herself because of his mental illness, but that day she couldn't hold back.

I'm sorry Ma, stop hitting me. Please Ma, stop punching on me. I bust my as for you and your siblings and this the thanks I get. I'm trying to keep a roof over yall head and you out here selling drugs while I'm at work. Anything you do in the dark will come to light Donnie. It's only a matter of time before your ass get caught. The street life ain't for you. You ain't built for that. You ain't sharp enough mentally, to be running with those boys. They're ruthless Donnie. If you mess up their money, they gone fuck you up boy. You out there playing with your life. I raised you better than that. I could lose my job behind your shit. You lucky your little black ass still a minor, you would've been out on the streets. Them ain't your friends out there. They gone have your little handsome ass right in prison. They like good looking boys like yourself in there. They try to make you their girlfriends. Unt unt. I don't play that. You won't have a choice. You can't fight the whole prison. They say the guards be in on it too. You keep going down this route, you'll find out real soon what prison is all about if you don't change your life. I ain't going to prison Ma, you ain't gotta worry about that. I'm almost 18. I'm gone be ok. Oh, you got it all figured out now huh. Alright know it all. We gone see. Don't be calling me from jail. I don't condone that kind of behavior. You brought shame to this family Donnie. I raised you to be a man and work for what you want. You know you were on thin ice with me from the jump. I hate to do this, but Tommy gotta go. I warned you Donnie if you did anything out of character, he had to go. This was way left field and definitely out of character for you. When you get felony convictions on your record Donnie, it's going to be hard to get a decent job or a place to live. After you get out of jail from doing your time, the felony follows you around for life. It's never ending. People judge you on your past.

Gary G. McDonald

You're going to be homeless and letting the system to take care of you. They give guys fresh out of prison, food stamp cards and assistance like someone living pillar to post. That's not what I want Ma. I don' want to be homeless and I don't want to be on welfare. I don't want the government doing nothing for me, Donnie said with authority. I was selling drugs to help you. I'm tired of seeing you struggle. I don't see anyone else trying to help you. I was trying to be the man of the house Ma. Boy don't be raising your voice at me. I'm sorry Ma. There's no reason for you to be out there hurting your community with that poison. God don't like ugly. I'm not ugly ma. I'm handsome right? That you are Donnie. Your ways are ugly. The things you do are ugly. Not you per say. Get it? Yes ma'am. I brought you into this world, and I can take you out. Get out of my sight boy. Go to your room. I don't want to see your face until it's time to eat. And probably don't want to see it then either. And as a matter of fact, get that dog out of my house immediately. He's no longer welcomed in this house. Tell Tommy how you messed that up for him Donnie. It's freezing outside Ma. I'll take him out first thing in the morning. I don't want him to die. Just get it done knuckle head. First thing in the morning. No exceptions. You lucky I can't get rid of your little black ass you would've been going with him. The law says I gotta take care of you until you're eighteen. That's not far off. Sorry I got you kicked out Tommy. I'll find you a good home. I won't leave you out on the streets. Boy I heard you went to jail, said Bryan. What your little ass did? Bryan asked. Five -O jumped out on the crew and slammed us all to the pavement. They found dope on me and took the boy to Juvie. Mom came and got me and now I'm home. Ma making me get rid of Tommy, said Donnie. It's your own fault. Ain't nobody tell you to get caught. Five-O caught yall slipping. Damn I fucked up bad this time. You know somebody that will let Tommy stay with them? Nah little brother. I found my own place by the way. So, let Tommy come stay with you for a little while until I figure things out. I have a few dollars to give you for room and board. Man, Tommy ain't finna be cockblocking my pussy. Scaring females away and shit. I'll pass little brother. Be safe Donnie. Catch you on the flip side. Tell Tay and John I said bye. Ma got my address. Yall could come by and visit if you'd like. We're getting older Donnie, everybody gonna start needing their own space eventually. We can't stay kids and live with Ma forever. Now you on the other hand, you might be around for a while. You not ready to have your own place no time soon. It's a lot of responsibility to have your own place. It's a lot of bills and thinking that goes into it. It's not just living there, it's other things that have to be done. I love you little brother, take care of Ma dem. If you ever need me don't hesitate to call. Ma got my home number. Bye bro. Bye Bryan.

Handsome

Chapter 6

Gang Related

The next morning Donnie did as he was told. Before going to school, he went to a fellow gang members crib to tie Tommy down until he came back.

Thanks bro. I'll be right back after school. No problem, fam says the gang member.

Daniel hurries along to school before he's marked absent.

Hi, sorry I'm late Ms. Smith, it won't happen again. I told you last time if you were late that you were going to detention. I was only a few minutes late. Can you let me slide this one time Ms. Smith? Please? No, you may not.

The class starts to laugh at the back and forth between Donnie and Ms. Smith. Donnie got frustrated and slapped papers from his teachers hand.

Now that's three days suspension. You want to make it seven? Fuck you Ms. Smith! Donnie shouted. That's seven days. Bye Mr. Prince. Go to the Principal's Office now! I'm sorry Ms. Smith. Too late for an apology Mr. Prince. If you're getting trouble in school, imagine what you're going to be doing in the grown up world. A bad attitude will put you in a few places you don't want to be. Like the graveyard. Or prison. I hear you ma'am, but don't talk me to death. Thanks for the lesson on attitude. I'll cherish this conversation forever. Like I said, Principal's Office. See you later Ms. Smith, Donnie says jokingly.

Donnie walks to the Principal's Office with pride, as he's given a seven day suspension.

Now I could hit the block and not worry about school. Shit! I forgot. Ma wants me to quit the gang. She must don't know, ain't no getting out. It's death before dishonor. Blood in, blood out. They ain't finna kill me. I gotta go home and check the answering machine. I know the school left a message by now. At least I got Tommy, he'll never change up on me. These voices in my head driving me crazy. I wish they would stop. Fuck! God pleased help me. Take these voices out of my head. They're keeping me up all night. Please help me. Amen. 82015100

Daniel leaves school and walks to his friends house to get Tommy. Upon his arrival to get Tommy, a rival gang member spots him and wants to start trouble. Donnie sees his rival and throw up gang signs.
      Gary G. McDonald

The gang member spins the block and pulls out a gun and starts shooting. Donnie runs in between two buildings, nearly being hit by a forty caliber bullet. The rival gang member speeds away in a lack box Chevy.

Damn that nigga tried to kill me. Jesus Christ! Let me get my damn dog. Tommy what you doing boy? You missed me? Let's go make some money.

Donnie walks back to his block where his crew is selling dope. They greet each other with gang signs and handshakes.

What's up yall? Man, I got suspended from school. I was wondering why you was out here so early, said the big homie. That school shit for the birds. If it wasn't for my mama being on my case about it, I wouldn't even go. That's real O.G. We ain't gonna use none of that shit in real life anyways. Well probably the math part and reading, but not the rest of that shit, said Donnie. I feel you lil Donnie. You a sharp little motherfucker bro. Smart dudes need to stay in school. The block ain't what it's cracked up to be, said the O.G. All of this shit a trap. A cat and mouse game. But when you're hungry, you ain't got no choice. You feel me? Yea O.G I'm listening. Being out here will land yo little ass in jail or the graveyard. Ain't no in between jit.

While Donnie's sitting there talking to the O.G, he starts fidgeting and looking around. He forgot to take his meds and began acting erratic. The O.G was side eyeing him, wondering what the hell was going on. Donnie tied Tommy to a fence and removed his shoes. He ran full speed to the stop sign and back. That went on for a few minutes, before being to put to a stop by the O.G. He was stunned by Donnie's behavior and have never seen anything like that on the block.

Lil Donnie stop bro! You good fam? You acting mad weird yo. You making me nervous fam. You seem a little off yo. You need a lift to the crib?

Donnie was sweating profusely and unsure of where he was. His eyes rolled in the back of his head. The O.G was panicking and didn't know what to do with the lil homie.

C'mon bro. I'm about to take you home. You got people stopping and looking over here. You gone make the block hot. Let me get your dog and put him in the whip, and I'm dropping yall off. You on any type of medication bro? I'm thirsty. I need some water O.G. I'm thirsty. I'm thirsty. I'm thirsty. Bro chill out! I'm gone shoot yo lil ass if you don't calm down. Get in the car yo. You blowing up the spot. You can't be out her if you can't control yourself. Get right. Then you can come back.
                              Handsome

I can't have you out here fucking my business up acting all weird and shit. You feel me? The O.G asked. Money over stupid shit fam. You still one of us Donnie. No sweat. Just take care of yourself. We're here to you crib Donnie. Get your dog and go get some rest. You're not doing to well bro. Handle that. I'll see you later.

As the O.G's pulling off, Bryan pulls up in his Honda Civic.

What's good O.G, O.G? Bryan asked. What's wrong with your brother youngin? Is he bugged out or what? I like the little nigga and all, but he can't be out here having fits and shit. I had an uncle like that. He was unpredictable as fuck. Your brother can get fucked up like that, or worse. I'll handle it O.G. My bad bro. I ain't know he was out there trippin. He was taking his meds O.G. I should've come by and warned you guys about his mental illnesses. But he loved the crew like family, Bryan said cautiously. Illnesses? How many does he have? He suffers from bi-polar disorder and schizophrenia. Whoa! That's heavy youngin. Make sure he's good before he come back around here, then we'll talk. Alright O.G . Thanks for bringing him home. No problem Bryan.

Donnie you Ok? I'm thirsty Bryan. I need some water. C'mon, lets go in the house.

Bryan grabs his brother and escorts him into the house. Donnie stumbles into the front door and is still unsure where he is.

Ma, you here? Bryan asked. Tay, you here? Why you yelling? What's going on? Tay asked. Donnie had an episode out on the block with his crew. The O.G had to bring him home. He was mad and embarrassed that Donnie showed out on his real estate. The CVL's don't fuck around, said Bryan. Drink this water bro. Here. Open your mouth and take this medication.

The O.G drives back to his corners and tells the crew that Donnie's not welcomed back up there unless it goes through him. He was an outcast until further notice. Ain't no posting up or cracking jokes from here on out. Bro got a lot of mental shit going on. Aight O.G, we on it. Get the word out to the rest of the crew. He ain't right upstairs. He looks normal, but he ain't. I'll get the word out boss. Alright. Get back to your spot.

The O.G was very cautious about ever letting Donnie back on the block. In fact, he was thinking more like indefinitely. Donnie had already gone to jail and came up short once, and never repaid his debt, so it was hard for the O.G to let that slide. His mental illnesses saved him for the time being. Normally if the gang felt that you were a liability, they would simply pop your top, but he O.G was cool with his brother Bryan.

Gary G. McDonald

Days later, Donnie returned to school and apologized to his teacher for his outburst. That same day, The O.G was also given an apology for him wilding out on the block. He was told not to come up there anymore, but it was Ok if he stopped by and spoke. The O.G wanted Donnie's dog for his troubles. Donnie started to tear up, but he knew that if he said no, his body would be stretched out on the sidewalk. Donnie handed Tommy over to the O.G. He bent down and hugged him, whispering in his ear, promising to get him back. Donnie walked off crying and beating on his head in frustration.

I'll be back for you Tommy, don't you worry. That's fucked up how he took my dog. I ain't scared of the O.G. Who does he think he is? I need me a gun. I'm going to get my dog back. Fuck the O.G. I'M BOUT IT! I'm ready to go all out about Tommy. That's the only thing I have that cares about me, besides John and mama. Nobody else in this family cares about me. The voices in my head talk to me more than my own family do. That's sad. It's cold as hell out here! I can't leave Tommy out here to be raised by the O.G. He ain't gone treat him right. He ain't gone treat him like I would. He probably won't even feed him. Ma trippin. That's fucked up, she making me give my dog away. I'll never forgive her for this one. All the times she had my back, and now she doing this to me. She broke my heart with this one. I can't believe that she would do this me. I should wait until it's dark and go steal my dog back. The O.G might kill me if he catches me, but I don't care. Shit! He might kill my whole family too. I can't let them suffer because of me. I gotta deal with this shit on my own.

Donnie walks home enraged at his mother and the O.G that muscled him for Tommy. He walked home slowly as he contemplated on going back to start some shit. The voices in his head told Donnie to pop off, as one of the voices of reason told him to chill out. There was always a constant battle going on in Donnie's head between good and evil. Although growing up, his mother always said that prayer changes things, Donnie was beginning to lose faith in those words. He's been praying and asking God to help him since he was a child, and nothing has worked. The voices told Donnie to walk in front of a train that was coming his way. He was aware how much that would hurt his mother, so he fought off the impulses bestowed upon him.

I am the captain of my fate and the master of my soul. I am the captain of my fate and the master of my soul. I am the captain of my fate and the master of my soul. I am Invictus.

Handsome

Chapter 7

N.A.M.I

Established in 1979, The National Alliance on Mental Illness have been offering their services to those who need it. Millions of Americans, regardless of race, creed, or color are affected annually with mental illnesses. These illnesses can be combatted with intense therapy, followed up with taking their medications. For many, the stigmas surrounding mental health, makes it difficult for people to come forward and get help. There are warning signs loved ones can pay close attention to if someone having a mental break down. Excessive worrying, constant fear, confused thinking, mood changes, prolonged feelings of anger, loss of sleep, difficulties understanding others, hallucinations, avoiding friends, lack of insight, thoughts of suicide, misuse of pills, drugs or alcohol, and physical ailments without cause can be some early signs that we can detect. Many of these mental illnesses can be overlooked and passed off as bad behavior early on with children, such as being hyperactive, nightmares, temper tantrums, aggressive behavior, poor school performance and being disobedient. In most cases parents are reluctant on getting help for their child out of retaliation and being labeled slow or retarded. Children now are being pawned off for a disability check with no signs of real mental illnesses. Regardless of age, don't be afraid to reach out and ask for help. N.A.M.I has a national prevention hotline at 1-800-273-8255. As of 2021 there are no test that can accurately diagnose anyone that has mental illnesses. Professionals use what's called a DSMMD, which stands for Diagnostic and Statistical Manual of Mental Disorders to evaluate patients. The manual includes a list of criteria that must be followed, such as time limits and behaviors to be classified as having mental illnesses. When dealing with someone that has mental health illnesses, it's important that they have health insurance. Doctor visits, treatment, medications and living facilities can be very expensive without the proper coverage. Most private insurers don't cover things involving mental health. If they did, the premiums would be astronomically high. Obamacare, Medicaid, Medicare, Chip, or Tri-Care are free or little to no cost for an individual or loved one if they qualify. If you or someone you know suffer from mental illnesses, it's not going to be an overnight fix. It takes a lot of hard work and commitment to stay on track, but with mental illnesses a person can easily get derailed. That's why N.AM.I has mental health professionals across the globe to keep you on a straight and narrow path. There are five steps in helping to find the right mental health specialist for you or a loved one.

Gary G. McDonald

Step 1 is to think about whom you're looking for. Step 2 is to gather referrals. Make sure the providers will cover things you need to have done. They have mini medicals and discount plans that pose as traditional insurance just to make a commission, so be extremely careful when selecting an insurance provider. Make sure you ask them on recording or have them put it in writing that they cover mental illnesses, facilities and medications. Try to get at least three names and numbers of providers with your specific needs. Step 3 is making the call. Don't procrastinate. If need be, have a family member or a friend to get the ball rolling for you. Step 4 is to ask questions. If there's something you're unsure of, just ask. The dumbest question is the one you don't ask. Step 5 is building relationships. Trusting people are major factors when someone is seeking help. Sometimes the first person you see, might not be the perfect fit for you. Keep it moving. There are more professionals in the sea that would love to help and want the best for you. Relationships can suffer surrounding the stigmas and misunderstandings associated with having mental illnesses. Good relationships can provide love and stability when a person is feeling lonely, sad or depressed. Whereas bad relationships tends to worsen things. People that suffer from mental illnesses have things that trigger them. Knowing what those triggers are, could save you a lot of time, arguments and money spent on a judicial system that has no compassion towards them to begin with. Being a hundred with your partner and telling them about your mental stability may not always be the best approach. Things like that takes time. As the relationship builds and grows, then you can consider thinking about opening up further. At some point, you would want your partner to know exactly what it is that they are signing up for, instead of them going in blind. What people don't know can get them hurt, or worse, if it's not presented properly. Hurt people hurt people, and in most cases, people suffering from mental illnesses don't know that they're inflicting pain. They don't know about the nights loved ones are up worried about them. These days and nights of despair can turn into resentment and being ousted by family members or a lover. The sandwich strategy is effective when trying to communicate. Putting bad news in between two slices of good news, can help calm emotions and ease fears. If a crisis arises, they have Crisis Intervention Teams that can assist if one is in the area. The N.A.M.I helpline at 1-800-950-6264 can help you with support and the right resources to get you through troubling times, or email them at info@nami.org Mental illnesses are conditions that affects a person's thinking, moods or feelings. These illnesses are anxiety disorders, bi-polar disorders, eating disorders, post traumatic stress disorders, depression, schizophrenia disorder, borderline personality disorder and obsessive compulsive disorders. Doctors have a number of treatments for a variety of disorders, but ultimately, it's up to the patients to take them. When a person dealing with such illnesses forgets to take their meds or does it on purpose, it affects everyone around them.
Handsome

It's a sensitive topic that's being widely discussed today, and the more we talk about it, the sooner the stigmas surrounding it will go way. Psychotic medications influence the brain chemicals that regulate thoughts and emotional patterns. Over the years doctors have prescribed a number of medications used to fight their illnesses, such as Camprel, Adderall, Saphris, Xanax, Abilify, Stattera, Zulresso, Rexulti, Sublocade, Suboxone, Wellbutrin, Vraylar, Celexa, Klonopin, Pristiq, Cymbalta, Ritalin and a plethora of others to help patients keep or gain control of their lives. Certain things can be the cause or symptoms of mental illnesses, such as smoking, selfharm, sleeping disorders, thoughts of suicide and substance abuse. With continuous therapy and a commitment to taking their meds, they can get control of what's happening in their lives. Police will be called out less. There will be minimal interactions between the police and someone having an episode.

Charlamagne Tha God over the years has used his platforms to spread awareness and the stigmas that surround mental health. His New York Times Best Seller "Shook One" has helped countless of viewers and listeners confront their own issues and open up about the topic.

For years we've all been guilty of calling someone crazy, schizo, looney toon, retarded, slow, bugged, or can't get right. These words are harmful, mean, hurtful and can be triggers for those dealing with mental illnesses. By shedding light on the subject and bringing a national awareness to it, more and more people have been seeking help. If you or anyone that you know are suffering in silence, you're not alone. There is an entire community dedicated to getting you the assistance and resources available in your area.

Contact N.A.M.I national prevention hotline at 1-800-950- 6264

Gary G. McDonald

Chapter 8

CAn't gEt RiGhT

Men, women, boy and girls suffering from mental illnesses don't see the world as we do. A lot of their irrational and erratic behaviors are forgotten once the chemical imbalance is in check. Time heals all wounds, but not for everyone. Those that have gotten caught up in the midst of an episode, will never forget how they felt at the time, or how they were mentally hurt by it. To a person living with mental illnesses, it's just another day in the neighborhood for them. Life isn't going in the same direction as they are.

Years have passed and Donnie's been in and out of jail on numerous charges. He'd also manage to father two kids after several bids in prison. The CVL's banned Donnie from hanging on the block and stopped everyone from associating with him. The O.G said he was bad for business. He was no longer affiliated. The rejection caused Donnie to wild out even more. The niggas he hung out with, bust heads with, sold dope with, fucked bitches with no longer wanted him around. Donnie was undoubtedly upset but didn't give it anymore energy. Instead, he decided to go play some basketball at a local park. Things were going great until Donnie caught a sharp elbow to the ribs. He immediately figures the guy wanted to play dirty, so he gave him a taste of his own medicine. Danny knees his opponent in the back of his calf and gives a jab to the kidneys.

What the fuck yo? You alright bro? Nigga you elbowed me. What's good? Donnie asked. Stop crying like a little bitch and play ball, said Donnie. You don't want none of this bro, Donnie says as he pounds on his chest. Man fuck this game, I'm Out of here. Man, you are weird bro, says the ball player. You act like that nigga on the movie Life, Can't Get right, the ball player says jokingly. Man fuck you and fuck this game.

Bystanders watch and laugh as the ball player teases Donnie on the court.

Don't run now Can't Get right. Give me a straight up fade. I'll beat yo ass. Matter of fact, I'll beat all yall ass. Fuck this bullshit ass game. Yall just mad I was going to dog walk yall on the court. Keep that ugly ass orange ball. Fuck yall. We gone miss you Can't Get right the ball player says loudly.

He knew that I was going to blow him out on the court, so he turned on me. Let me go home before I fuck a nigga up out here. Who got next? Donnie asked. I do. Can I run with you bro? Nah I got my team already.

Handsome

Just say you don't want me to play with you. I don't want you to play with me, says the guy on the sideline. Bro you really showing out. Are you ok fam? You off your meds or something? Fuck you and stay out of my business, Donnie shouts. I need a job. I need to make some money. You know someone that's hiring? Hey, are you ok bro? You need me to call someone for you? I'm fine. I'm waiting for my dog to walk up. You hear him barking? Donnie asked. Nah bro. I don't hear anything. You bugging out fam. Anybody got a cigarette? Bro you should leave. Somebody gonna call the police on you. Fuck the police. Fuck fuck, fuck the police I'm coming straight from the underground, a young nigga got it bad cause he brown. It's not the other color that some police think, they have the authority to kill a minority, but fuck that shit I ain't the one to a punk motherfucker with a badge and a gun to be beating on and thrown in jail, we could go toe to toe in the middle of the cell. Fucking with me Cause I'm a teenager wit a little bit of gold and a pager. Bro this nigga singing N.W.A. What the fuck yo? Get your cousin off the court fam, he's losing his marbles. The police killed you yesterday homie. How are you here playing ball today? Donnie asked. Fuck them and the police. Bro, just leave, I don't want them to fuck you up, says the guy on the sideline. You're off bro. Go home and take your meds. I know the signs fam. I got peoples that be bugging out like you. I'm trying to help you. I don't need nobody's help. I can take care of myself.

Police were called to the park about a disturbance on the basketball court with a mentally ill man, in his late twenties, early thirties, wearing blue gym shorts and no shirt. Donnie continued walking back towards his home when he was stopped by Chicago Police squad cars.

Hey. What I do officer? Put your hands on the car Sir. We were called about an altercation at the park with a black male fitting your description. Where are you coming from boy? I ain't no bot, I'm a grown ass man with rights. Why am I being arrested? I'll do all asking questions. Do you have any drugs or weapons in your possession. Nah, I ain't got no drugs and weapons. I was at the park playing ball. This some bullshit officers. I ain't do shit. Yall always fucking with black people. I can't stand yall son of a bitches. Sir why are you sweated so badly? It's hot as fuck out here and you have me on the hood. Your ass would be sweating too if this was you. Oh, we got a wise guy, the officer says as he continues to pat Donnie down aggressively. I bet yall sorry asses get a kick out of fucking with black people. You cowards scared of us. We put fear in yall hearts. Yall crackas to come to work clutching your guns out of fear. Pussy! Take me in, I don't give a fuck. They'll give me my medication and I'll be back on the streets. Stop resisting! I'm not I'm just standing here, said Donnie. You're going to jail for resisting arrest and drug paraphernalia. Resisting and drug paraphernalia? Cracka you gotta be shitting me. I ain't got shit on me. If I do, you put it there. Fat ass cracka. I hate yall. You got to lie on a nigga to lock him up.

      Gary G. McDonald

That's sad. This how yall meet yall quotas huh? Locking up black people. We helping yall pigs fill up your jails. All of these privatized prisons yall own. We know all about it. Motherfuckers out here buying prisons and being promised that their beds will be 70 to 90% full. We up on game in Chicago. I don't know about the rest of the world, but we know what yall up to. Do you get extra credit or points for shooting and locking up black people? Be honest officer. Do you ever shut up? Your mouth stay running. Geesh. You should've been a lawyer, says the officer. It's never to late. I could become one on jail. Hell, I could even be Mayor or commissioner too with a felony conviction. I bet you didn't know that officer. I could be your boss someday. Have you seen my Pitbull Tommy? He's beautiful. I named him after my brother that died. Did you see him? Donnie asked. Can he come to jail with me? We left him out on the curb with your other dawgs. We even gave him some dog food and water. Ok? Thanks officer, that was nice of you. Don't mention it kid. How long have you been able to pay attention? Huh? What's your name Sir? Donnie. Donnie what? Donnie Prince Sir. Well we're taking you to the 13th Precinct. I need to call my lawyer so that I could sue for harassment. My momma know people. She's a bus driver, she has a lot of connections. Can I have some water please. I'm dehydrated officer. You'll be ok, we're not that far from the station. You could drink all the water you want. Just sit back Donnie boy and enjoy the ride. You have priors, so you know the routine. Can you drop me off to my mother's house officer? We can't do that. I'll lose my job Donnie boy. Then I'll be pissed at you for it. That's when I'll shoot your black ass, the officer says jokingly. Can you call her and tell her that I'm going to jail please? She's going to be worried and think something happened to me. Something did happen. You wilding out at the park and caused a scene, now your going to jail for it. I didn't harm anyone. This is absurd. What's your badge numbers? If she know people like you say, she probably already know your black ass going to jail. Yall got a village, right? Everybody know everybody business, right? You damn niggers always trying to politic yourselves. You need the police around. Everybody keep screaming defund the police. If we weren't around it would be more murders, robberies, rapes and break ins. We are the peacekeepers, despite what you blacks think, Donnie boy. That's not my name officer. It's whatever I want it to be boy. You don't get to call shots here, that's my job. I'm the shot caller around her. Now if you keep popping your chops, I'll be inclined to give you additional charges. That's what pigs do right? They oink. Oink Oink pig. You ain't shit cracka. Let me call my momma real, quick. I'll be nice from here on out. I have mental problems officer. I need to see a doctor. I don't need to go to jail, I need the proper help. They have medications in jail too Donnie boy. Don't you worry. They're going to take good care of you and your brain. Ok? Yes Sir. We're here. You could tell the nurse all about it. I'm sure she'll get you what you need. I just need to see a doctor, please. He can't get right. You need a doctor to think for you? That's just God awful.
Handsome

You need to ask for a new brain like the scare crow on the Wizard of Oz, there Donnie boy. Goddamn can't get right! I love that damn Martin Lawrence and Eddie Murphy movie Life. I be tickled pink. Those sons of bitches have me laughing so hard, I be about to piss my pants. I watch that sombitch whenever it's on tv. That damn can't get right hit that ball to the bushes. Passed them damn trees out yonder. Can you hit a ball like that too Donnie boy? You could get your family out of the ghetto if you can. I'll hit yo ass with that ball pig. Fuck our racist ass, Donnie shouted. C'mon, this is your new home. Now I gotta add another charge for threatening an officer. You niggers show make my job easy, and I get overtime when I have to do paperwork. I love my job. I was supposed to be getting off, and now you saved the day. Plus, I don't have to go home to my nagging wife. I should be thinking your black ass for this, but I won't.

After I'm done with you, the Judge will be rushing to send you ass off to prison. Your kids will think that you're a scumbag and don't give a shit about them. They'll grow up hating you for not being around. Even your job will think you abandoned them. Even if you get out, they ain't gonna want to hire someone like you, that talks to themselves and don't know left from right. You're a liability Donnie boy. You can't be trusted. You're too unpredictable. The only place for you to go is jail or live in a mental facility. I bet you don't have a girlfriend either. I told you, you can't be trusted. You might have a knife up to their throats for all they know. Who wants to take a chance on someone unstable?

It's dangerous shit Donnie. Your mom might even be tired at this point and ready to put your grown ass on the streets too. The world goes on Can't get right, whether you're in it or not. The world keeps spinning. Time don't stop either. If you don't want to stay here forever, don't be sassing no white officers. I don't care what you do with your own kind, but you gone respect us Donnie boy. Doing the opposite gets you a one way ticket to hell, jail or a better place. It's your decision on how you would like to live the rest of your life.

Shit or get off the pot. You follow me Can't get right? Do you understand the words that are coming out of my mouth? I love that damn Chris Tucker from Rush Hour. Yes Sir, I do. Thanks for not killing me like the rest of your buddies be doing to my people. You racist as fuck, but you cool at the same time. You should be a comedian when you are off duty, said Donnie. Yeah, yeah. I'll think about it. I'm taking off your handcuffs, don't try to run Donnie boy. There's nowhere for you to go. I'm going to have them call a nurse down here to evaluate you. Good luck. Whatever.

My momma will have me out of here in no time. Damn it smells like ass in here. I hate this fucking place. They brought me here for no fucking reason.
      Gary G. McDonald

Chapter 9

Suicidal Thoughts

Suicide has been a way of preserve a family's honor in Asian cultures. The Samurai saw it as a code of honor. In America, it's frowned upon. It's considered a sign of cowardness and weakness. Someone, that life was to hard on and they felt as though, God put to much on them that they could bare. Or it could be a person suffering from depression, post traumatic stress disorder, anxiety, insomnia, sleep apnea or a myriad of other illnesses that can cause someone to take their own life. Making attempts can be a cry out for someone that's lonely, sad, depressed or looking for attention. That attention can be from parents, a lover, a guardian or something they don't like about themselves. An adult or a child that had traumatic experiences such as childhood abuse, war traumas, and sexual abuse are at high risk of suicide. Someone that is threatened with prison time, bullying, finances, academic failure, the loss of a loved one, or the end of a relationship. Most of those losses, failures and mishaps can be recovered from, by a person that's thinking rationally. A person suffering from mental illnesses aren't thinking as clearly as you and I are. They might be handsome, beautiful, sexy, fine or gorgeous on the outside, but on the inside there's something that can be dangerous to themselves or others. Looks can be deceiving, and sometimes it's hard to tell if someone is thinking about taking their life. Especially if they're not opening up about it.

Hey Donnie boy, get used to your new home, you're going to be here for a while. You threatened an officer. This ain't my home, Donnie said angrily. I live with my mother brothers and sister. I bet you ain't got no family. You probably can't even make kids. You shooting dog water. You pissed your pants watching Life. You're dumber than I thought, said the officer. I'm smarter than yo mama. Get him out of my face nurse. Adios Migos. You're mad at the wrong person. You mad black people was here first. We're the original people. Yall mad because we could stay out in the sun all day. White people on a timer. Tick tock tick tock. It's vitamin D for us. It's skin cancer for yall, Donnie said jokingly. Yall gone burn up in the sun. It's vitamin D baby. Your friends at the basketball court called the police on you, white people didn't do that, said Officer Karen McVee. Open Cell number 2, said the C.O. Get him down to the infirmary and have them do an evaluation. The way you're acting, you're lucky to be alive, said officer Karen. Me personally I would've just shot your ass and got paid time off. No trial. No grand jury. Plus, I'm a white female. What jury would convict me? It's called qualified immunity. Look it up in the law library on your leisure time. You know what leisure is Mr. Prince? I didn't think so.

Handsome

Stand your black ass up boy. I ain't your boy. My name is Donnie. I bet you'll understand a boot to your face huh. You know that language well huh Donnie? You want me to call back up down here for you? The way you're looking at me makes me nervous, said the C.O. Maybe I should get the K-9 Unit in here and have his dog sniff all in your ass to see if you got any drugs in your rectum. Got anything up in there Donnie? That's how yall smuggle it in ain't it? Nah, the C.O's bring that shit in. Yall be in here raping niggas too. I bet yall wives don't know yall like boys. You mouthing off to me boy. Stand down officer, he waiting to see a nurse. He's not all there. He don't understand what you're saying to him. I'll take it from here said the Sgt. Thanks Sgt. Can you get someone in here to bring me my meds please? He told me to take my own life. If I die, I'm gone haunt him in his sleep. I'm gone be right there to scare the living shit out of him and his family. You can't keep treating black people like this and not have any repercussions. You ever seen Tales from the Hood? Those little black slave dolls attacked the governor. That shit was too funny. On earth yall the big bad wolf, in yall dreams, we run shit. All the lives yall steal from the world, coming back to get yall, Donnie said laughingly. You got jokes huh? We'll see how funny it is when your black ass don't eat. You're all ours. Nobody can help you here. You're a danger to society. You need to be in a straight jacket. I'm gone see to it that you're in a padded room. You might try to hang yourself, so we're taking your clothes too. You'll be cold and naked. Willie Lynch said to break you like a horse. You got to tame niggas and show them who where the pants around here. Months gonna go by before the public defender gets to see your case. You sassed the wrong officer. Man, I don't care about you or anything you talking about. Hey Johnson, this one wants to kill himself. Put him in room by himself. I ain't say that, you're lying on me. God ain't gone leave me in here with yall pigs. God don't like ugly, nor filth, and this place is both.

As Donnie hoped and prayed, a crisis team from N.A.M.I was dispatched to get him out of custody and into their facility for treatment. When the team had arrived, Donnie was still irate and wasn't making any sense. He was belligerent towards the staff and the officers and had to be quickly sedated to deescalate things. Donnie woke up some time later and was thoroughly evaluated then sent packing. His mother and sister came to pick him up from the facility and immediately drove him home, while saying a prayer for her son. Day's later after Donnie's release, his brother Bryan was killed in a drive by shooting. Two of Mrs. Prince children were dead and there were only three left. She got tired of questioning God and fell into a deep depression. Mentally drained from work and the deaths of her son's, Mrs. Prince took another paid leave of absence to make funeral arrangements and to wrap her head around things. In Donnie's mind, Bryan got hit up because of something he did, and the guilt was beginning to rattle his cage.

Gary G. McDonald

It's my fault that Bryan's dead. It's all my fault, Donnie shouted. Bro, this has nothing to do with you. He was at the wrong place at the wrong time. A few people got killed that night, not just Bryan. Things like that happen when you're living that lifestyle, said John. I promise this had nothing to do with you or your mental illness. Stop being hard on yourself. Have you taken your meds today? I took them earlier. Thanks for asking. I'm just making sure. First Tommy and now Bryan. I don't need something happening to you as well. I can't lose all of my brothers. Who's going to be out here to have my back? It feels like God punishing mama because I'm like this. This ain't got nothing to do with nothing Donnie. You're reading to much into this. I ain't ask God to make me this way, she did this on her own. I'm a good person, right John? I should be normal like everyone else. When you pray at night, could you ask God to fix me? I got you bro. I'll tell him tonight before I go to bed. Thanks John. If mama a good person, that take us to church, pay tithes, cloth us, and feed us, why God keep giving her bad luck? I don't think it's fair. Momma gone end up like me. It's too much for her. I thought bad luck was for bad people. I ain't know good people could have bad luck. Life's too confusing. Are you going to miss Tommy and Bryan? Yeah, I already do. The house is too quiet. Things will never be the same. Even though he had his own place, he was always at our house. He couldn't get enough of mama's home cooked meals, said Joe. It won't be the same around here, that's for sure. You think we gone see them again like people be saying? I hope so. I'll be sad if I never saw them again, said John. I want to see them again. I wonder if they gone be older or younger. Do people get old in heaven? I don't think so, according to the Bible, they don't. Mama gone be sad for a long time. Parents not supposed to outlive their kids. I still think it's my fault. Nd my dog gone. The police left him on the corner. This shit ain't right John. Now it's just the four of us. We a two man crew now. PB2, Donnie says jokingly. You think mama gone stop loving us because they died John? Nah. Why would you think that? I don't know, I was just asking. I think she'll love us the same. It's just taking a toll on her because it's back to back. She ain't had time to fully heal from Tommy's death. You worry to much Donnie. Just don't be asking her things to irritate her. I know that you might think that you're helping but go easy on the questions. Try not to mention their deaths. Let her rest and gather her thoughts. She don't need any extra stress right now. Ok? Alright big bro. I won't bother mama. I'll be quiet. Now, go get dressed for the funeral, before Ma kills us too. Then she'll be lonely. I don't think she'll kill us John. I was joking Donnie. Don't worry about it, just finished getting dressed. We can't be late. How are your kids doing? John asked. Little man good, he's getting big as hell, and so is his sister. Their mother always trying to hit me up for child support like I'm rich or something. I got to get me a good paying job. I need me a doctor or a lawyer girlfriend that got some cheddar. I'm trying to wife them asap bro. I'm an asset around the house. I could fix things and lay pipe, Donnie says jokingly.
       Handsome

You got to have some duckies in the bank. They don't want a broke man. You need mula, and dinero to bag a professional woman like that. It takes more than looks and dick to keep them around. They only date working men, drug dealers, ball players and professionals, then comes the lowlifes after they've been hurt a thousand times. If you're broke, they're losing. They're going backwards. I guess you're right, said Donnie. Seeing his brother being lowered into the ground, reminded Donnie of Tommy's funeral and how it gave him the chills. Donnie's inner voices were beginning to taunt him.

It is your fault. Your brother doesn't know what he's talking about, the voices said. You and only you are to blame. You should've been the one in that casket, not Bryan. Your brother was shot by the police, protecting you. They killed him. You should make them pay. No, the boys at the basketball court did it. Everybody's guilty. Kill everyone. Nobody's to be trusted. Your dog Tommy probably did it. Side eye everybody. If you're blaming yourself, you should take your own life. Yeah that's what you should do. Do it Donnie! Do it! Nobody will miss you anyways. Do it! Kill yourself. Do it! Join your brothers in heaven or wherever they are. C'mon, do it scaredy cat.

After the funeral was over, Donnie rushed to the upstairs bathroom to get a straight razor to slice his wrist. Oh my God Donnie! Why you did this to yourself bro? C'mon Donnie, mama going through enough, and now you pulling this stunt. This will send her over the edge for sure. Clean up this mess before she comes in here. We got to get you bandaged up. If she see those cuts, she's gonna freak out. I want to go where Tommy and Bryan at. If you kill yourself, who am I going to have here with me? I ain't gone have nobody to watch over besides Ma. I'm the protector of the family. Well at least I try to be. You still got Tay. That's different. Tay ain't you. You're my favorite and always have been. You know that. This will break my heart Donnie and mama's too. We're family. I can't lose you like this bro. We got to stick together. I always had your back, no matter if you was right or wrong, I had it. I need you around Donnie. Don't leave me bro. Be strong. Don't let those voices get to you. Block them out. It's easy for you to say, you don't hear them all day and night, I do. Ma needs us Donnie. We can't leave her in a time like this. She'll surely have a nervous breakdown if something happened to you. It'll be selfish on your part if you did that to our mother. You're right John. I'm sorry John. I don't know what I was thinking. These voices keep telling me to do all sorts of bad shit. I'm trying to fight them, but they're constantly bullying me. They have more power than I do. I have three voices telling me to do things. Two of them are mean and one of them is nice. They argue amongst themselves then turn on me. I hate it here! It's scary sometimes the thoughts I have, or they put into my mind. Don't tell mama I tried to kill myself. Continue taking your meds and do your best to fight those demons. I love you Donnie.
               Gary G. McDonald

Chapter 10

Neutralization Through Felonization

Slowly but surely, black and brown people are being neutralized by felony convictions. While we're out working, being productive citizens, raising our kids or shooting the shit under a tree, white supremacist and the powers that be are plotting to keep us stagnated. They want us right where they want us, living in poverty and at each other's throats. Our living conditions, the lack of education, crime, and PTSD from neighborhood shootings causes children to live in constant survival mode. Felony convictions are being handed out to black people like candy, while our white counterparts are given a slap on the wrist, misdemeanors and probation. The two America's we live in separates color along with class. Somedays it feels like no matter what we do or how hard we try to show them a different side of black people, we're still looked as a threat. Hell, it's written right there in our constitution that we're less than three fifths of a man. So why would white America see us as something different right? Now take those same thoughts, and apply a person suffering from mental illnesses to the equation. The outcome will be catastrophic. They believe it's a part of their job description to beat our asses and patrol the streets like predators. They're the sharks and overseers of black neighborhoods. The colonizers of the world, patrolling black communities with bad intentions. Shipping our family members from plantation to plantation, through felonization is the wave of neutralization. It's all premeditated. Separating father's and mother's from their kids, leaving them to fend for themselves or possibly molested in foster care. The court system could careless about your home life or what you want to become in the future. Their intent is to make you pay fines, inconvenience hard working people of color that make mistakes and continue to take. Enough is never enough for a well built money machine. An evil timeless, calculating machine designed to drain you of everything, even some of your freedoms. A machine designed to break the toughest of the toughest. Strong enough to bring a grown man to tears. Staring over from scratch makes you feel worthless. It seems like a long road ahead, but it can be done. Black people are being extracted from society on purpose. You can climb up the ladder of success as high as it goes, and they'll still find a way to put you into the system. It could start out as simple as a traffic ticket. If you miss a court date or don't pay the fines, now you have a warrant for your arrest. Now, that misdemeanor has the potential of gaining strength and becoming a felony conviction. It can seem like a never ending story. So many of us have been in the system or know someone that has. It's no joke. They keep you trapped. The walls are constantly closing. The jail doors are forever revolving. The streets of Chicago are ruthless, and any given day you could catch a bullet from the corner boys or the cops. Take your pick.

Handsome

Trying to get back at either of them could cost you your life or freedom. Systematically, everyone is against us. We're the bottom man on the totem pole. The race everyone loves to hate. With felony convictions, finding a place or a good job will be almost impossible. The more felonies you obtain now, the worse your life can be in the future. Donnie and the rest of us found out the hard way, by doing stupid shit to trick ourselves off these streets.

By the time Donnie was twenty five, he had been to jail more than twenty five times. Most of those offenses were drug related and due to his mental illnesses. Many of us find it hard readjusting into society and living productive lives because of over 170 disparities we face daily. Now add mental illnesses to that. They don't stand a chance. It's ten times worse for them. When you get locked up, you have to take your psyche meds, and now you're on everyone's radar. Either to pimp you out of your medications or to con you into doing something else in exchange. However, you swing it, you're a target. Homosexuality also plays an important role in prison and can be profitable for the inmates or all parties involved.

Donnie has never had an easy going jail or prison sentence. There was always fighting of some sort with the officers and the inmates. This time Donnie was in there on burglary charges and was serving a three year sentence. Donnie toned down his attitude and took his medication as prescribed and started to take baking seriously. He would bake some of the best bread and cakes for the C.O's, and word spread around the compound. Only a few months int his sentence and Donnie has found his niche. Manley Academy had only taught him so much, the rest he learned from the streets or in jail. Inmates would come across cookbooks and different recipes to try to get Donnie to make their favorite dish. He was starting to get used to his new, found fame until one day he didn't take his meds.

Donnie's notoriety was short lived as the inmates one by one began to turn on him after finding out he suffered from mental illnesses. We've all heard stories in the hood about a crazy person killing people and getting off. Like, they only had to go to a mental hospital for a while, with little to no jail time. That's what scare people. The unknown. Not that they don't like people with mental illnesses, but can they truly hurt you and get away with it, is most of their concerns. It's hard to decipher if someone is being them authentic selves. People that live with mental illnesses have learned creative ways to hide their secret. No matter how hard they try to conceal it, or contain it, eventually it will make him or herself known. Mental illnesses will always make their way to the surface, you just have to be ready when it does.

Gary G. McDonald

Chapter 11

Dear Mama

You alright bro? You're sweating bad. Here, have some water. The nurse should be here shortly. You was doing your thang on them cakes, then you smiled and went down, said an inmate. Them niggas over there laughing and shit like it's funny. Thanks for having my back bro. I really appreciate it. People treat you funny when they know you ain't wrapped to tight. I got family members going through it too. I've seen it all before. Nothing surprises me anymore. If you need a shoulder to lean on bro, I'm here for you. Thanks bro. I ain't perfect, and neither are they. Shit happens you know. I was born this way. You preaching to the choir bro. Thanks again for understanding. I have something to smoke, you could hit it later if you like to. You should get your girlfriend to bring some shit in for you, says the inmate. I'm single. I wish I did have one, she'll be bringing all kinds of shit in here for me. I got whatever you need. We don't need her. Not taking my pills snuck right up on me. Them niggas could've easily caught me slipping. I wasn't finna let nobody try you. I won't forget this bro. What's your name anyways? Donnie asked. They call me Tony the Tiger. Ok. Tony the tiger, good looking.

Momma's baby, daddy maybe. Mother's have been holding things down at home for millions of years, as well as business, agriculture, architecture, and you name it. They're natural nurturers that hold special places in the hearts and souls of every child they've given birth to. Carrying a child for nine months takes patience, determination and the willingness to want to bring a life into this world, with or without their father present. Not to mention countless of doctor's appointments they have to go to. Mother's are the backbone and driving force in society today. They could have one of the worse kids imaginable and will still go to bat for them. A mother's love stretches far beyond the eyes could see. It's infinite. It's magical. It's intuitive. Where would we be without mama?

It was a cold Thursday morning in Chicago, and Donnie's name was being called for a visit. Nobody has ever come to see him in jail unless it was his children's mother. He didn't have money to make 3-way calls, so he baked and did odd jobs to earn money to survive. He was shocked to see that it was his brother John coming to see him. It had to be something really bad for John to visit his brother in the freezing weather. As Donnie was being led into the visitation area, he noticed a look on John's face as if he had been crying.

Donnie immediately goes into defense mode, thinking that someone did something to his brother.
                              Handsome

What's good John, everything alright? What you doing here? The C.O gave you shit in the waiting area? Nah bro, nothing like that, John said as he teared up. So, what is it? Spit it out bro. What's wrong? Donnie asked with an attitude. Mama died Donnie. What bro? What? Mama dead bro? You serious John? What the fuck yo? My mama dead bro? Mama John? Donnie asked loudly. Say it ain't so? Mama ain't coming back bro. Sorry to give you this news while you're locked up, but I thought you should know. She's in a better place now, with Tommy and Bryan. I tried to go, and you stopped me. Now she's there before me. This shit ain't fair. I'm finna go crazy in here John. Now it's just me you and Tay. God must really hate our family John. Why else would he keep allowing us to go through all of this pain and suffering, Donnie cried. Calm down over there, inmate, said the C.O. Man my momma died, FUCK YOU! I ain't scared of you. I'm ready to die. Now I really ain't got shit to lose. The one person outside of you John that gives a fuck is gone. I love you bro, but I feel like I have nothing left to live for. My life sucks. I'm always in and out of jail. I'm fucked in the game.

The C.O hits the alarm and calls for back up. Donnie squares up as John pounds on the thick bullet proof glass for him to calm down. John begs for his brother to stop, but by then the C.O's fill the visitation room with riot gear. They form a line and stand one behind the other, with the one officer in front holding up an electric shield. C'mon motherfuckers, I ain't scared of yall. My momma just died, I'm ready to see her and my brothers. I'm ready to dance with the devil, Donnie shouted. Lets dance.

The C.O's rush in to subdue Donnie as he puts up a struggle against 6 correction officers. He was tasered twice with no affect. Nurses had to be called in to sedate the strong young man.

I want to die! Right now. Take me. I'm ready to meet my maker, Donnie said with a slurred speech. He was taken to the infirmary for evaluation, and later put in the hole for sixty days. Donnie laid there in an empty cell, wearing a hospital gown thinking about his family and how much he misses them. As he paced back and forth crying, he thought about the Tupac song Dear Mama. I reminisced on the stress I caused it was hell, hugging on my mother from a jail cell. And who'd think in elementary, HEYY I see the penitentiary, one day running from the police, that's right, my momma catch me and put a whooping to my back side. Fuck! I wish I could go to the funeral and see her one last time. I'm sorry I couldn't be there for you mama. You probably died from a broken heart. I'm sorry I gave you all of those sleepless nights mama. Forgive me. Tell Tommy and Bryan I said hello. I miss yall. Until we meet again.

Donnie worked out intensely during his sixty days on lock down. He wanted to be physically fit and ripped just in case someone stepped to him.

Gary G. McDonald

It was hard for Donnie to get the deaths of his family out of his head. He wanted to get off some of the built up anger that was brewing inside of him. He thought about taking off on the first C.O he saw but didn't want to get any additional charges. So instead he settled to knock out an inmate. He felt that would make him feel better about the death of his mother. As Donnie patiently waited for the doors to be opened, his temper had calm down and he had changed his mind about fighting. He later signed himself up for anger management classes and an early release program. Donnie was adamant about changing his life and getting a handle on his mental illnesses. For the next two years, he took his medication regularly and earned certificates in both cooking and anger management classes. He was ready to re enter society as a productive citizen. Weeks later, Donnie was released, and John was there to pick him up from jail.

Thanks for picking me up bro. No problem Donnie. I wanted to run something by you little brother. Oh ok, shoot. I got a job offer out in New York and I'm seriously thinking of taking it. You should move up there with me. John suggested. Do we have any family up there? That's along ways from here, Donnie said worriedly. I don't know about this one John. New York though. It's just as worse as Chicago. All of our family is here. What family? John asked. It's just me, you and Shante. Everybody else gone bro. You won't be missing a thing. We could fly back if you'd like and visit their grave sites, but it's done here bro. You gotta think about your future from here on out without them in it. We can't turn back the hands of time, we could only go forward. We've been here too long. Change is good. I want to see the world, not die here from a stray bullet or for wearing the wrong colors. That's no way to live Donnie. Just come with me bro. You'll live with me and I can keep you safe. I love you little brother. Mama made me promise to be my brother's keeper, and I'm sticking to it, John said with authority. You and I have always been the closest and I don't want to leave you behind. It's not safe out here for none of us, especially you. I can take care of myself John. Thanks for the offer, but I'm good right here in the City of Brotherly Love. Alright Donnie, I tried, I won't push. If you change your mind let me know. I'm not moving yet. I still have to get back with human resources to discuss pay and other particulars. Big timer huh? Donnie asked jokingly. A little something something, John replied. My big brother moving on up in the world. You can too Donnie. You got to want better for yourself. Nobody can make you want it. It has to be in you. John said sternly. This old as Toyota about to overheat. I'm glad we're almost home. I almost forgot. I'm going to put the house up for sale. After the deal is done, I'm giving you and Shante yall portion, and you could do whatever you like to do with your money. Spend it wisely Donnie. I'm taking my share and putting down on a place in New York.

Handsome

Mama gone flip over in her grave if you sell the house, Donnie said worriedly. Where am I going to live? Have you thought about that Mr. businessman? I have Donnie. That's why I want you to come with me. I don't want you out here wandering the streets with nowhere to stay. I don't want somebody sticking a knife in you because they don't understand your illnesses. At least with me I know you'll be safe. Man, people get killed everywhere, New York included. So, you just gonna leave me here? That ain't love John. You're abandoning your favorite brother. First Tommy. Then Bryan and now mama. This life doesn't seem real. I feel like I'm in the Matrix. Life ain't worth a fuck. I'll survive though. I'm built ford tough. Remember? I remember Donnie. I'm the on who said it. Could you run me by Gold Bloom Baking. Somebody in prison said they were hiring felons.

I gotta put in an application asap. I was the man in prison. I had the kitchen on lock down when I wasn't on lockdown. After the car cools off, I got you bro. If you continue taking your meds regularly, you could live a decent life Donnie. People don't know you have a mental illness until you forget or neglect to take your medication.

They're looking at your handsome face and body structure, then boom, the erratic behavior. It's only so much you can get away with using your looks. Attitude is the other part of living a good life. That's the part you have to control. Once you get that down pack the rest should be a breeze. I'm afraid to leave you here, but I have to better my life. I feel like Chicago's holding me back.

 I feel like I'm drowning here. There seems to be more opportunities for me there with my field of expertise. You don't have to make up your mind today, just consider it little brother.

Donnie goes in the house and take a good hot shower before going to put an application in at the bakery. He takes a long look in the mirror and smacks the sides of his head so that he could focus. I will survive this. I will survive this. You're stronger than you look Donnie. Focus. It's just you now.

Gary G. McDonald

Chapter 12

Inner Demons

Man shut up! Just stop talking, Donnie shouted. Get out of my head damn it! I can't get out of your head, I'm apart of you. Everywhere you go I go. The only difference is, people can see you, they can't see me. I'm just a voice in your head. Your thoughts are also my thoughts. Don't you get it? My name is Peter, just in case you were wondering. I wasn't wondering. I want your ass gone, said Donnie. I've been taking my medications regularly and I can still hear you. What's the sense in taking this shit? Why you asking me? I'm you. These are questions you should be asking your doctor. If I were you, I'll throw them all away. Or better yet, take all of them at once. Look at you sitting here talking to yourself at work. People can hear you Donnie Boy. Don't call me that. I'm ignoring you from here on out, said Donnie. That's impossible, Peter replied. Try it and see how that works out for you. You're wasting your time. Keep talking out loud, people will surely think you're a crack pot. Remember, they can't see me or hear me, Only You can prevent forest fires Donnie Boy, Only You, Peter says jokingly. If you kill yourself, I'll go away. That's the only way to rid yourself of my insanity. Just like the gang you used to be in. You lucky they let you leave with your life. They must've felt sorry for yo crazy ass. Blah blah blah, I can't hear you, says Donnie, as he puts his hands over his ears. Look at how you look. People gone think you're a loon. I'm scared. You shouldn't be mean to Donnie. I like him.

We're all alone Donnie. Mommy's gone, so is Tommy and Bryan. What are we going to do without them? Who are you? Donnie asked. I'm Roman. I'm the nice voice. You're a chump, just like Donnie Boy. Two pussies, Peter shouted. You're a pussy Donnie whispers. Come say it to my face, Donnie Boy. I wish I could you son of a bitch. You're scared of me, that's why you're hiding in my head. Come out and show yourself, Donnie shouts. Ahh, shut up, You, ain't gone do shit. Put your thumb in your mouth you mam's boy. Or better yet, put in in your ass. You're pathetic. I'm surprised that you haven't killed yourself already. You're so draining and depressing, you make me want to shoot my ownself, said Peter. Only a mother could love a son like you. I hate when you speak, it's irritating as hell. Donnie get rid of Peter. Get rid of all of us. Have you taken your meds today? Donte asked. No, I forgot to. Well brace yourself for some ups and downs today. Don't mention it, said Donnie. Today going to be one of those days. It's important that you take your medications Donnie. That's why you can hear us so loudly. I don't like how they make me feel. I start gaining weight and feeling like a zombie. I hate that feeling.

Handsome

Roman's too weak for this crowd. He's always wining about something. You're to soft to be around us. You're the weakest link Roman, goodbye. Get your little silly putty ass on about your business. This here for grown men. Your kind ain't welcomed here. Yall both need to shut up, said Donnie. It's time to take my meds, hopefully it'll quiet the both of you down. If I could stop yall ass from poppin up, it's a wrap. You can Donnie Boy. It's only one way. You know how to do it. Do it! Do it! Do it! SHUT UP! Donnie screamed, as he took three pills at once. Hopefully this shut yall up for good. I hate noise, Donnie said with hostility. I'm with you until the end Donnie Boy, like Chucky the doll. My buddy, my buddy, everywhere I go, he goes, my buddy, my buddy and me, Peter says jokingly. I'm just having some fun. Don't take me serious Donnie Boy. You should unscrew your brain or take one to the head. It's a good day for a suicide. Don't listen to him, he's evil. Shut your pie hole Roman, before I kick your ass. Your raining on my parade here. I don't need you twisting Donnie words around. I can't wait until this medication kicks in. Yall blowing my high. Are we driving you crazy Donnie Boy? I need some peace and quiet. Could you shut up please? Can you believe the nerves of this nigga? Peter asked. I should make you stick your hand in the oven. You ain't gone do shit to me Donnie whispered to Peter.

Hey Don, can I speak with you for a minute in my office? The supervisor asked. Yea sure. You see what yall done did? Now I'm in trouble for my outburst.

Donnie walks over to his supervisors office and takes a seat. He sits down nervously, hoping that he didn't lose his job.

Hey Donnie. What's up boss? You know that I like you and all, you're one of my best bakers, but I can't keep having the outburst. This is a drug free, professional environment, says his supervisor. People are starting to talk. I don't care what you do on your private time, or how you are outside of these doors, but while you're here, I need production and less drama. Is that clear Donnie? Yes Sir, crystal clear. I apologize for that. It won't happen again. This is your second warning. The next time it's a write up, then a suspension and after that, it goes in your file. Write ups keep you from getting promotions and advancing in the company. Nobody wants to stay in the same position with the same pay forever. Do you want a raise Donnie, or do you want to stay right here? I want to get promoted Sir. If you have Tourette Syndrome or something, try your hardest t control it. We like your work, you're a hell of a baker. Man shut your ass up, Donnie ain't trying to hear all of that yapping, said Peter. Don't talk us to death cracka. We don't need this job. You sound like you want Donnie to beg for this shit. Fuck this dirty ass job Donnie. You should slap that cracka in his mouth and throw your apron in his face.

Gary G. McDonald

Flip this desk over bro. You scary as hell. You just going to let him talk to you like that and get away with it? Peter asked. You ole soft ass, Tiny Tim ass nigga. You're pie as fuck. Your heart pumps cool-aid, Peter shouts. Don't listen to him Donnie, Keep your job. Don't panic. It upsets me that he's doing this to you. We should cry together, said Donte. You're a real square. Kill that idiot Donnie. I keep trying to tell you that he's the weakest link.

Thanks for the opportunity and the vote of confidence. I love my job and what I do here. I'm an asset to the company. I'll do better Sir you have my word. Alright Donnie, you can get back to work now. If all goes well, I'll be able to throw some overtime your way. I appreciate that. Thank you, Sir. No worries. Just don't make me regret it, says the supervisor. I won't boss. Why you just ain't call him a sorry son of a bitch? What's with all of this boss shit? You know what it really stands for, Peter says jokingly. Ain't that's what boss means in prison. I thought you were tough. You scared of that skinny ass dude. You're lame Donnie. You ignoring me can't get right? You ignoring me boy? Peter says in a rednecks voice. You can't ignore me forever. You speak back eventually. Blah blah blah blah blah, Donnie whispered. You trying to make me look crazy? Donnie asked. That don't take much effort. You're supposed to do what the voices tell you to do. Not the other way around. You suck Donnie. Don't pay him any attention. He's bored and miserable, said Roman. He an attention seeker. You should cry and worry that your job is in jeopardy. Aren't you sad that your family is gone? You have to cry and let it out. Don't suppress your feelings. You can always be real with me Donnie. I don't judge or make fun of you like that voiceover Peter. He's a bully. He's going to get you fired. You'll be homeless. I might be sad, depressed and cry a lot, but I'll never try to send you to prison. I got your back Donnie. I wish the both of you would disappear for good.

The workday was coming to a close, when Donnie noticed a few of his co workers pointing fingers and talking about him. Peter wanted him to step to those fools. Donnie remained calm and kept his composure.

See you guys tomorrow. Thanks for giving me a ride home Sheila, I really appreciate it. The guys at work been acting funny. They act like we're back in high school. You know why right? Sheila asked. No why. Somebody put it out here that you be talking to yourself and that you might be schizophrenic. Wow, we all talk to ourselves, said Donnie. That's human nature. What makes me different? They just mad all the girls be talking about you and not them, Sheila says with a smile. Oh really? What they be saying Sheila? You know, shit like, he's handsome. I wonder if he got a girlfriend. I bet he packing. He's so fine, yada yada. The usual stuff women talk about. Umm, I see. Slice her throat Donnie. She probably be over there talking bad about you too, says Peter.

Handsome

She ain't shit bro. She's toxic. You should hop out of the car while it's moving. You don't hear me talking to you? Answer me damn it. You should grab the steering wheel and cause yall to wreck out. She probably talk more shit than a little bit. Are you ok Donnie? You got quiet on me over there. Sorry about that. I was thinking about my mother and brothers. She passed away when I was in prison. I didn't get to say my goodbyes. It still bothers me, that's all. That's understandable Donnie. Well if you're free this weekend, I wouldn't mind doing something fun. All I do is work and go home to my seven year old son. Motherly duties huh? Is his dad around? No. He rather run the streets and hoe hop. He ain't trying to be a family man. His homeboys are more important. His dumb ass could care less about his child. God will get him on his own time. Enough about him. Are you taking me out this weekend or do I have to go out alone? Sheila asked. I would love to take you out. You're beautiful and you got a nice body. Do you exercise or are you just fine in general? Meaning, are you naturally sexy? And you have a car to get us to dinner, I'm all in Sheila. How can I say know to that? It's a date then, Sheila replied. Indeed, it is beautiful. I'm so excited. I haven't been on a real date in some years. Most guys want to come by and have sex, and don't mention courting you. Not saying that I'm a virgin, but it's more to me than sex. You get it or nah? I understand. I used to be the same way when I was growing up and didn't know any better, Donnie said jokingly. I'm also a private person. Can you keep our business between us? I don't want people at work questioning me about the time we spent together. If they weren't there, it's their loss. I'm really looking forward to seeing how you are outside of work Sheila says in excitement. Everybody always talking about you, now I get to see for myself. I'm a little touchy feely too sometimes, I hope you don't mind. No, I don't mind. Do your thing. I'm affectionate myself, Donnie says as he caresses her thigh.

Donnie's strong hand grips Sheila's leg, as she began to get turned on by it. Back and forth he rubs in between her thighs, giving himself an erection. His third and forth fingers, finally bends inward, cuffing the print of Sheila's pussy.

You know what you doing Donnie? Of course, I do. Do you like it? Donnie asked. Yes, Sheila says in a faint voice as she tries to focus on the road. Ok ok, we're to your house. You got me all hot and bothered. You sure know how to turn a girl on. I hope you're even better at finishing. G whiz, you have my panties soaked Donnie. I ain't been this horny in a while. You really got me looking forward to this date now. I was just about to say I can't wait to tell my girlfriend about it, but I'm gone wait until things get a little more serious before I jump the gun.

Sheila shakes her head and looks down in between her legs, then gives Donnie a hug and a kiss on the cheek. See you later handsome. Alright.
Gary G. McDonald

Chapter 13

Speed Dating

Yo what's good Donnie? Where the hell you been at? I ain't seen you in a few years bro, said the homie from the CVL. I've been in and out of jail. They can't keep a good nigga down, said Donnie. The O.G told the crew a while back that nobody was to talk to you because you was bugged out. Yeah, I fucked up in front of the O.G. I apologized for it though. He said I was straight, but I couldn't come back up there. Hey, you got some of that "Love Boat" on you? Donnie asked nervously. Yeah. What you need? The homie asked. A twenty is good, said Donnie. Aight, bet. Stay right here. I'll be right back.

The dealer runs through the alley to his stash and quickly emerges with the dope. Donnie looks at the baggie and gives it a flick with his finger. He's content with the product and gives his ex-gang member some dap.

Good looking fam. It's the weekend and I'm trying to get high, real high Donnie said with enthusiasm. Alright Smokey, the homie says jokingly. Don't get fired on your day off. That's some powerful shit there. You act like I'm new to the game. I don't need you to school me, Donnie says disrespectfully. Aight bro, it's time for you to step. You getting out of character.

After copping his dope, Donnie headed back home in a hurry hoping not to get stopped by the police. His inner demons continued to taunt him as he walked with drugs in his pocket.

You better hurry up, Donnie boy. If they catch you this time, you're getting fifteen years. There they go! Peter shouts. Where? Donnie asked. April fools sucker. I tricked you. Fuck you Peter. I hope this dope can get rid of your stupid ass. I'm tired of your big ass mouth, said Donnie. I hope it gets rid of all of us. Let's overdose together Donnie Boy. Do the whole twenty. Put it all in a needle and take off. Don't smoke it. The high ain't the same. Beam me up Scotty. I'm ready to see what's on the other side anyways. Get out of my fucking head! Donnie shouts. I ain't going nowhere. Make me leave fool. Closing your eyes won't get rid of me, you gotta walk into traffic for that. That'll put you out of your misery for sure. Be quiet, Donnie shouted. I'm not even real. I already told you that you're the only one that can hear me, besides Roman scary ass. Be quiet asshole. Why should I? You created me. You can make me go away too. I can't wait until you go on that date. I'm gone fuck your shit all up. Sheila will never go out with your black ass again after I'm done with her. People at work gonna be talking again after she tells them about your conditions. If I were you, I wouldn't go Donnie. He sounds serious. I believe he'll do it for real, says Donte.
Handsome

Everyone at work gonna know about you. Your secret will be out. You won't be able to hide that shit for long. When you throw that drink in her face, she's really gonna flip out and beat your ass. Black women don't go for that these days, but I'll get your stupid ass to do it. SHUT UP! SHUT UP! SHUT UP!! God please stop him from talking. God can't hear you. It's only me and the devil. We control you. God don't like people with illnesses like us. I think it's funny to him. It's all a game. I think he despises your family. Look at how he treat yall. Everyone's dead Donnie Boy. Get high and catch up to them. I'll go with you, Peter said happily. You should just do yourself in and do us all a favor. The world would be less one person with schizophrenia. If those girls knew you were a gook, they wouldn't look at you twice. Your mother left you and so did your brothers. Nobody likes you. They're running away from your ass to the other side. You're driving the people around you insane. It's rubbing off on your friends and family like a plague. That's not true. People do like me. I'm worthy of being loved. I'm a real person and you're not, Donnie shouts. Don't be getting loud with me Donnie Boy. I'll make the police catch you right now. I can make you do or say anything that I please. I OWN YOU.

Donnie finally makes it to his place and immediately rolls up a laced joint of weed and speed (PCP). Knowing the effects of the powerful drug and what the aftermath can look like, Donnie continued to puff away.

You done went and done it now. Ain't no turning back from this one Donnie Boy. If I were you, I wouldn't do drugs. It can kill your brain cells and us. Donte said worriedly. I'm grown. It's the weekend and I'm trying get high. Period. Yall find something else to do. Be gone. Donnie shouted.

Donnie fires up his joint again and feels amazing. The voices in his head had rattled him so badly, he forgot that smoking wasn't allowed in the basement that he was renting. The renter smells something foul coming upstairs and bangs on the door for him to stop whatever he was doing.

That shit is stank as fuck! Put that shit out. You know the rules Donnie. You're being disrespectful towards my house. I have children that live here, the renter shouted. I'm sorry Ms. Johnson. I had a rough day at work. Excuse my manners ma'am. It won't happen again, Donnie yells loudly. It better not, or you'll be looking for a new place to stay. Sorry Ms. Johnson. Mann, fuck Ms. Johnson! Peter shouted. Who does she think she is talking us like that? You should walk your scary ass up there and give her a piece of your mind. Go up there and let her know exactly how you feel. If I were you, I would bash her head in. I'm not listening to you Peter. Don't do it Donnie. You're smarter than that, said Roman. He's trying to trick you into going to jail for life. Block him out Donnie.

Gary G. McDonald

Let me think. Stop talking. I have a date in a few hours. Roman, try to keep Peter quiet for me. If he messes up my date I'm screwed. He's stronger than me, I don't know if I can. He'll get me. You can do it Roman. I have confidence in your ability to shut him up. Worry him to death, Donnie said as he continued to prepare for his date. I'll try, I can't make any promises Donnie. I'm high as hell. Now I'm hearing another voice. Shit! I shouldn't have smoked. Fuck fuck! I should cancel and just go another time. Nope. Don't try to back out now you coward. You rubbed her thighs and got her pussy all moist, and now you want to stand her up. She won't give you a second chance. You see how fine she is? This your only chance Donnie Boy. Other men at work will be trying to get her. You better make an impression, said the Boogeyman. Where did you come from? Donnie asked. You created me just now. You don't remember? We should go out and scare some people. We should have a serial killer on the loose in Chicago. What you say Donkey? My name is Donnie. Whatever. Donnie, Donkey, there all the same, said the Boogeyman. Let's go out and make a few white women clutch their purses, and a few niggas nervous. Nah, I can't do that. I ain't trying go to jail again. I'm done with that shit. You're done when we say you're done. We OWN you Donkey. I'm trying to get dressed you perverts. You ain't even take a shower. You smell musky, the boogeyman said jokingly. Damn I forgot. If yall shut the fuck up, I'll be able to concentrate. It's too much noise in here. I need quiet, Donnie shouted. Yall can't all talk at once. We can sing together but not talk together.

Donnie took off his clothes and got into the shower. The effects of the laced joint was beginning to kick in. The hot water was starting to feel like acid on his skin. He was trippin hard and had only minutes to get dressed before Sheila showed up. The higher Donnie felt, the quieter the voices had gotten. For the time being, they didn't seem like an immediate threat of ruining a wonderful evening. Minutes later, Sheila had arrived and bumped the horn to alert her presence. Donnie was nervous and sweating profusely. The PCP laced joint had him on GO. His eyes were bulging, and his mouth was dry from being dehydrated. After getting dressed and spraying on some cologne, he got a paper towel and wiped the sweat from his face and bald head.

Hey beautiful. Sorry I took so long. You're looking good. Thank you handsome. You clean up nice yourself. So where are you taking me? Sheila asked. To hell if you don't pray lady, says the boogeyman. I thought that I'd treat you to a nice seafood restaurant. Are you allergic to seafood? No. I eat everything. Seafood is my favorite though. The food there is awesome. You'll love it. Where is it? Sheila asked. Keep straight and make a right at the light. You smell really good Donnie. What are you wearing? It's called Aramis, Donnie replied. You're full of compliments tonight Sheila. I give credit where credit is due, she said.

Handsome

I see that. Look at Donnie boy acting all mushy. You sound like a square over there in the passenger seat. Why are you back? You should've been long gone by now. Can't you see that I'm on a date. Aren't you supposed to be in someone's head? Yeah yours. When you fix your brain, I'll be gone. Until then, you're stuck with my irritating ass. Whatever said Donnie as he sucks his teeth. Did I say something wrong? Sheila asked. Oh no, I had some food I my teeth, sorry about that. I was told that it was rude to do that, and I needed a toothpick. Yeah that would help, and it would be a little less intimidating, said Sheila. You're right, I'll practice at it. Practice makes perfect. I've heard that a lot growing up, Donnie said, as he started to sweat profusely. Could you turn the air up please. I'm hot. I'll fill up your gas tank. Is that better, Sheila asked. Are you nervous about something? I've been known to have that affect on men. That's much better. I appreciate it. The restaurant over there on the left, by the corner. Oh ok, I see it. I've heard a lot of good things about this place, but I've never eaten from here. I'm eager to see what it taste like. Good. First time for everything. I'm thirsty. I need some water. Some cold ice water would be great right about now. Are you ok Donnie? Yeah, I'm just a little hyped up. I'm like you Sheila. All I do is work. I don't get out much. That's how I'm able to afford this expensive dinner, I save my money. Aww. Everyone should treat themselves to a good time once in a while. The going to work and home routine gets boring after a while. You start to want some company. Being alone can drive a person insane, said Sheila.

They park the car by the front entrance. Donnie gets out and runs to open Sheila's door. She gives him a huge smile and says thank you. A little hesitant, and watching Donnie closely, they walk into the restaurant. He made sure that she knew that chivalry wasn't dead.

Thanks Donnie. You're a real gentleman. That was nice of you. You're welcome beautiful. Can we have a table for two? Donnie asked. Sure, right this way, says the hostess. Your waiter will be with you shortly. Ok, Thank you.

You look really nice Sheila. Your lips are juicy, your hair looks amazing, and you smell yummy. Boy you better stop gassing up my head, it's already big. Gone head with your handsome self. You gone be done got yourself in trouble. Trouble my middle name beautiful. Can't you tell? Donnie asked. Is that so? What kind of trouble are you trying to get in? Inquiring minds want to know Donnie. A penny for your thoughts, Sheila said jokingly. You ain't got to be quiet now. We're both consenting adults here. What's on your mind Donnie? I wasn't trying to be to forward, sometimes my comments come out nastier than intended, Donnie said nervously. I'm a big girl, I can handle it. I bet you she can. SLUT! She's trying to get fucked on the first date Donnie. That pussy belong to the streets. Or that damn bakery you work for.
Gary G McDonald

I bet her vagina is on fire right now. You should throw a drink on her to cool that bitch off. Ask her when the last time she had an STD test. Or ask her how many guys have she slept with in the last year. You don't deserve a good girl like that, I do. If I were you, I'd slap her in the mouth right now, Peter shouted. I used to get my hair done by your sister Shante some years back. She was always busy and had a bunch of hair and nails to do. I could never get an appointment. Yeah, she was good at doing hair. She works a 9 to 5 now. She still does it on the side when she has time. Hi, I'm your waitress Tiffany. Would you like to start off with something to drink or some appetizers?

What would you like to drink Sheila? A Hennessey and coke would be fine. And for you Sir? A Sprite for me. Ok, I'll be back with those drinks in a minute. I think I asked you earlier were you allergic to anything. Yea you did. I told you that I eat everything, Sheila replied. Pussy too? Donnie asked. What? Sheila asked, as she choked. I'm sorry, I don't know where that came from. My apologies. That's ok. To be honest, yes, I've played around with women before. I never went down on them and I never stopped them from feasting on me. That was in my younger, wilder days. After having my son, I grew up and put all of that behind me. I was fun while it lasted, until it wasn't. I'll say this, women can be very possessive when they want to be, Sheila says with caution. What about you Donnie. Nope. I've never been with a man. I got tried a bunch of times in prison though. Dudes was always calling me handsome and being extra nice to me. I used to see them doing it by their bunks and in the showers. I ain't gone lie, I watched a few times because that's the only entertainment we had in there besides sports and tv. Wow! TMI. What's TMI? Donnie asked. Too much information. I wasn't talking about you being with a man, I was talking about you eating pussy Donnie. You sure you ok? Your starting to act a little weird. Oh, I'm sorry. You was talking about you being with a woman. I thought you were asking, have I been with a man. It was a misunderstanding, said Donnie. I'm confused. Boo! Donnie shouted.

Everyone in the restaurant stopped and looked over at their table. Donnie was sweating like a hooker in church.

Donnie you're embarrassing me. Sheila said angrily. What's wrong with you? You're starting to scare me Donnie. Boo! Donnie shouts again. Boo! He shouts. If you don't cut this shit out Donnie, I know something. I'm gone leave your ass right here at this restaurant.

The white waitress felt something was wrong with the black couple sitting at table 2 and had her manager contact the police. As Sheila tries to calm him down, he knocks silverware and plates onto the floor. Sheila gets up and walks to her car in disbelief. She felt bad for her co-worker and didn't want anything else to do with him. He was arrested again.
        Handsome

Chapter 14

Never In, A Million Years

What's good bro? You're back already? Didn't you just get out? Tony the Tiger asked. Yea, and now I'm back. I guess you can't get enough of this place huh. I be having my fun here too. I understand Donnie. Trust me I do. Man, Life so fucked up. Every time I think shit good, it goes to shit again. It's like I'm always going backwards. I had a job, a place and a potential girlfriend. Now all of that's gone overnight because of this mental illness. I blew it. I swear a nigga can't get right to save my fucking life. Don't be so hard on yourself Donnie. We all have our ups and downs. It's not about how many times you fall Donnie, it's but what you do when you get up. At least you got a release date. I'm sitting here fighting a case doing day for day. You know what they say bro. You only do "two days". The day you go in, and the day you get out. You had a chance to do better in life, and once again you were dealt a bad hand. We all get the shitty end of the stick. Especially if you're black. We see that shit more than any other race. You can't let it break you Donnie. If you need to talk, you know where to find me. I'm just so disappointed in myself. I can't control shit. My mind be taking over for me and I have no control over it. That's scary as hell bro. Never in a million years I would've thought I would be back here, especially this fast. It feels like I was just in here the other day. Something told me not to get high before going on that date. But noo, I did it anyways. I'm too grown for my own good. Shit costed me everything, Donnie shouted. My landlord probably going to throw my shit out on the streets. Whoa whoa, calm down Donnie. I'm on your side bro. You a short timer. Don't end up staying longer than what you have to. You ain't got nothing but ninety days, you could do that standing on your head, said Tony. Small potatoes for a giant like you. You're right. I'm stressing over nothing. I need to stay focused. Thanks for the pep talk fam, I needed that. Ok, so when you jump, don't forget to send me my money for the consultation fee. I should reach out to Sheila, but she probably thinks I'm crazy and wants nothing else to do with me. These fucking voices will be the death of me. Somebody called? Peter asked. Oh God. Ain't nobody call you. Leave me the fuck alone. You're the reason I'm back here in the first place. If it wasn't for you and the boogeyman, I would've been laid up with my new girlfriend. Yall trying to purposely ruin my life, Donnie shouted. That's the plan, said Peter. I ain't did nothing to you. I just want to live in peace. That's all I ask. Let me live in fucking peace. That's all you do is yell, scream and talk shit. I'm sick and tired of it. Me too Donnie Boy. End this shit. End it now! Peter said aggressively. I wish yall was dead. You not allowing me to live a stress free productive life. I have so many felony convictions because of yall. I can't keep living this way. I don't know which one of you might pop out and try to assassinate my character.

Gary G. McDonald

You guys are too unpredictable. Without us, you'll be a boring lonely person. We keep you on your toes Donnie. We keep you active and feeling alive. Those pills make you feel like a worthless zombie. Yeah, we may say crazy shit, but at the end of the day, you created each of us. There's nowhere for us to go but up from here. They could only keep us here but so long, then we're free again, until you do some more stupid shit. Now you want to kill us. Impossible! You're wasting your time Donnie Boy. It can't be done unless you go with us. That's the only way. You created me, now deal with it. That goes for me too, said the Boogeyman. I'm not here to stress you out anymore than you already are, says Roman. You can get rid of me whenever you want to. I won't put up a fight. I'll be sad but I'll get over it Donnie. I'm not mean like they are. I want the best for you.

Donnie closes his eyes and places both hands over his ears an screams as loud as he could. He screamed so loud, it scared an officer and made him drop his coffee. He as immediately taken to the infirmary to get checked out by a nurse. Donnie's condition seemed to have gotten worse. Although he'd been taking his medications as prescribed, the inner voices were much stronger and louder than Donnie could handle. The voices controlled his every sense of being. No matter how hard he tried to block out the noise of prison life and his inner voices, the more difficult he found it to be. In Donnie's mind and the minds of millions of people suffering from mental illnesses, they think the switch can be turned on and off like that. Peter, Roman and The Boogeyman were there to stay. He couldn't shake them. They were with him every waking moment of the day. It was in jail when he finally realized that he was taking those voices to the grave with him. Donnie was once again released into the wild with nowhere to call home. Released amongst the judgmental and hypocritical, all pointing their fingers and gossiping like children. Acting like their shit don't stink. Pretending that they're not suffering in silence on the low. Putting on fake smiles and hiding childhood traumas wasn't possible for Donnie , like it isn't for many of you.

Man, where you been? You're like Houdini. One minute you see you, the next minute you don't, said Johnny from the 12th St Group. I know bro. I can't seem to stay out of jail. These pigs are always locking me up for something. I can't get a break. They're always right on top of me. You would think they'll treat people with mental illnesses with compassion. I think it makes them madder to be honest with you, said Donnie. When we don't respond to their commands, or if we don't understand what's going on around us, they get furious bro. They don't have the patience to deal with people like me, so instead they just lock us up. It helps with their quotas an keep the beds filled at the 70 to 90 percent capacity the private prisons are promised.

Handsome

You're always welcomed to hang out with us Donnie. Ain't nobody perfect. We have our faults too, niggas just ain't been diagnosed with shit. Sorry to hear about your mother and brothers bro. That shit ain't right. Life suck sometimes, said Johnny. Shit, for me and my family, it sucks often. The devil stay coming at us. He don't take no days off. It feel like the walls closing in on me Johnny. Its all about what you make it. Life's a bitch, then you die. I had a cousin that was always depressed and saying weird shit, we just learned how to deal with it. Then eventually, we learned to overlook it. He's still family, just from a distance, you know. If anybody fucks with him, they got me to deal with though. He don't bother nobody. But people be hearing him talking to himself and they start picking at him or throwing stuff at him. Shit pisses me off that he can't defend himself like a normal person would.
Are they hiring up her at the car wash? Donnie asked. Yeah, but it's a revolving door. They always hiring and looking for dependable workers. You can't be missing days and you can't be having no drama up here. The owners don't play that shit. Just do your job and keep it moving. If you're on any type of psyche meds, please take them before coming to work. I don't need you flipping out on me or the customers. It's my head on the chopping block for referring you. Don't let me down bro. Come by tomorrow morning and I got you. Thanks Johnny. Don't thank me yet. I owe you one. I appreciate you for hooking me up. Another thing Donnie, NO DRUGS. This is a drug free environment. No worries. I'll be cool. You won't have any problems out of me.

The next morning it was cold and sunny in Chicago. Donnie showed up to work promptly and ready to wash cars. Before the rest of the employees had arrived to work Donnie walked around to check the place out. Peter, Roman and The Boogeyman were all battling for position in the mind of a man trying to escape them. Deciding on who was going to take center stage at his first day of work.

Hey good morning Donnie. Are you ready to work? Johnny asked. Yeah, of course I am. Ain't nothing like making money. Did you take your spinach this morning? Johnny asked jokingly. Yea, of course bro. Never leave home without it. I hate how it makes me feel though. It slows me down and make me fat. But washing cars is like second nature. I could do it with my eyes closed, Said Donnie. I'm sure you can. The cars are already in line. Grab that bucket over there and fill it up with soap and water for me please. Alright boss. Donnie says condescendingly. Don't let him boss you around Donnie. Don't lose this job too, Donte said worriedly. Ignore him. Spray his ass with the water hose bro. He care too much about this dumb ass job, Peter shouted. Spray his ass Donnie Boy. Do it! BE QUIET! Donnie whispers. I'm thinking about building my own carwash. You gone help me bro? What you mean? Saving up money and buying you a carwash? Johnny asked. Yeah, that's what I meant. Nah I'm gone build it by hand brick by brick.
                          Gary G. McDonald

Donnie you're trippin yo. I told you yesterday, no weird shit. I'm gone build a big ass mega carwash, right over there. Donnie said confusingly. Where bro? Right there? So, what you gone do about that bank sitting there? You going to buy them out or have it knocked down? I haven't thought about all of that. I just know that I'm gone build one. Mann just keep washing cars yo. Don't be telling people about your plans. Keep them to yourself. Don't worry about the carwash right now, just focus on today. You said you wanted to work, so work. I did my part getting you the job. It's up to you to keep it. You promised you wouldn't be any trouble. You gave me your word bro. I did that, and I'm here. Are you sure you took your spinach? Donnie Boy, he's belittling you. Don't stand for that shit, Peter shouted. I told you I took it. Why you keep coming at me like that Johnny? You acting like you the owner. You right Donnie. My bad. Don't let him off the hook Donnie. Spray his ass with that water hose on purpose, by accident. I'll lose my job, Donnie whispers. Fuck this job, said Peter. You going to find me another one? Donnie asked. I got you Donnie. I'll find you one first thing in the morning. No, he won't. He's lying Donnie. Don't trust him, said Roman.

Donnie aims the hose in Johnny's direction and proceeds to drench his entire body with water. He was definitely off his meds and had smoked a joint before work. Johnny stood there emotionless as he contemplated on losing his damn religion. The patrons as well as their co workers were also stunned and left wondering if he was going to retaliate.

Bro you gotta go. You fucking up the first day of work. Oops. My bad Johnny. I can't help it fam. I don't know what came over me. I need this job. Please bro. I ain't mean to do it. Peter did it. Who? Peter. Who the fuck is Peter Donnie? You see a damn Peter over here? I'm finna go home and play Black Ops. You ever play Johnny? Can I come back tomorrow? I'm a good worker, and sometimes I'm not. Do you play Black Ops Johnny? I'm a good worker. Bro put down the water hose and go home before I call the cops. I'm really trying to be nice here Donnie, and as cordial with you as possible. Leave now bro, or you'll never be able to come around here again. You can't even get a carwash from up here you showed out so bad. Just leave Donnie, you causing a scene.

Donnie takes aim and soaks his old friend again with the water hose. He points it directly into the face of Johnny which sends him over the edge. The two men get into a tussle in front of customers. Punches were thrown from both sides. Police were dispatched and called out to the carwash and Donnie was arrested once again was later taken to the hospital for evaluation. Donnie was looked over thoroughly by a nurse as he continually mumbled twenty dwarfs took turns doing hand stands on the carpet. They couldn't get him to shut up about it. He repeated it for more than two hours nonstop.

Handsome

One of the doctors on duty overheard Donnie mumbling twenty dwarfs took turns doing handstands on the carpet. The words sounded very familiar to the doctor. His mind raced and raced through years of data and movies in a matter of minutes. He finally remembers hearing it from Warren Beatty's movie Bugsy Siegal. Who also had big dreams and suffered from mental illness. Because of his wild dreams of making the Flamingo Hotel and Casino a reality in the middle of nowhere, he was taken out. Donnie was released after being Baker Acted for seventy two hours. He wasn't sure if he was coming or going. Nobody was there to pick him up this time from the hospital. He's never felt more alone than he was feeling at this moment.

What the fuck am I going to do now. Another job, gone. Everybody dead. John moving to New York. My life ain't shit. Mama why yall left me? I don't know what I'm doing out here. I'm lost without you. Have you run into Tommy and Bryan yet? Why won't you answer me? C'mon mama say something. Please help me mama. I can't go on without you.
God if you let me talk to my mama, I swear I won't go back to jail. I need her guidance. We're here Donnie Boy. You see this shit? Everyone has abandoned you. What you feeling like now? I bet you feel like a pile of shit. Ha ha ha, that's funny. Let's go out and scare people, The Boogeyman said. White people always fucking with us like fuck with them. Let's put some fear in those motherfuckers. Ain't yall tired of their shit? I know I am. Me too, Peter shouts. I don't want to hurt no white people. I don't want to hurt anybody. I'm too scary for that. You got that right. You ain't never been down to do shit! Why you even here? Peter asked. You're way too soft for this bunch. You probably have on panties, Peter says jokingly. Wouldn't you like to know? Donnie get a knife and cut him out of your brain. He's corrupting you. You need to be the savage you are. Embrace that shit. He's right says The Boogeyman. Embrace it. Don't listen to Roman scary ass. He's not your friend.

Donnie walks towards the place he used to call home. The streets were jumping, crime was still happening throughout the city, and life was at a standstill for Donnie. The walls of the world and Donnie's collapsed heart was beginning to take it's toll on him. He wandered through the cold neighborhoods of Chicago with no money and no roof to lay his head under. A park bench was all he could find for the moment, as he reluctantly wanted to ask his siter for help. Donnie was at a crossroad on foot, with no resources and nobody to turn to.

Gary G. McDonald

Chapter 15

Twenty Dwarfs

These dummies can say whatever they want about me, but lowkey they really fear me. They won't say it in front of you, but they do, said Roman. I've been here since day one nurturing man's every desire. Your God kicked me out of Heaven simply because she was jealous of me. Can you believe that Donnie? I had more people following me than her. Just like you have followers on social media, it was the same there. Heaven's not a place Donnie. It's a state of mind. It's something that they tell every generation to control the masses. When you leave earth, you're not going to be living in the clouds. That's fairy tale shit. This heaven right where you at. Why you think the rich try so hard to keep what they have? They've created their Heaven, right here in hell. This is hell Donnie. So, my mama and brothers not up there in the sky? Donnie asked. No, they are not. Why should I believe you? Donnie asked. Who are you? This Roman, Donnie. Remember the one they're always calling scary? Oh yeah, I remember. Everyone has free will Donnie. You could ignore us and take your pills like you're supposed to, but you refuse. I only set the stage you pull your own strings. How many times have I tried to talk you off the ledge? Roman asked calmly. How many times have I shed tears with you Donnie? Answer me damn it! Roman shouted. That fear you walk around with, and those bricks you're carrying for your family will tie you down forever. The only thing that matters is the energy you create. Right now, you're full of a lot of negative energy. Hold on to that shit. Embrace the animal within you. Stop being a fucking pussy. Boss up Donnie. You sitting there looking like some ole pathetic mama's boy. Pull your fucking skirt down. Why do you think you're still alive. I have plans for you Donnie, but you're not listening, Roman shouted. I'm that dude Donnie. I rule this fucking earth, I just let you occupy space here. So, you're the Devil? Donnie asked in amazement. Where are your horns and red skin? Why can't I see you? Donnie asked. I guess Peter and The Boogeyman the devil too huh? No. They're my minions. They do my evil bidding. I'm very busy. That's why they're here most times. I only believe in God Roman. My mother always taught us about the horrors and evils that the devil is responsible for. She never told us anything good about him. Or you. Whoever said Donnie. Well she taught you wrong. I've been here for millions of years ruling the earth. God knows not to bother me. She lets me do my thing down here, as long as I don't impede on her kingdom or try to recruit her angels. I have millions of people to choose from right here. I can take my pic of different ethnicities, shapes, sizes, colors, religions. The "WORLD IS MINE"! Roman shouts. It can be yours too Donnie, if you follow my road to success where the niggas dress thorough and bitches say yes. God likes to watch. She's a jokester. She gives man instinct and other extraordinary gifts and sets the rules.
Handsome

Look, but don't touch. Touch, but don't taste. Taste, but don't swallow. You like to swallow Donnie? Roman asked. And while your stupid ass jumping through hoops and moving pillar to post, I swear, she's laughing her ass off. Not just at you, but at all of us. She's a tight ass and a sadist. She's an absentee landlord, Roman shouted. Everything I touch, goes up in flames. I can't seem to get right Roman. Why God made me like this? Why I can't function like regular people? Sins of the father Donnie. I'll leave it at that. The hand you're being dealt has nothing to do with you to a degree. Like I said, we have free will, Roman replied. I try to be a good person, but god keep allowing these voices to control me. No matter how many pills I take, or how many times I go to therapy, I still can hear them. It all seems like a waste of my time. I thought the pills were supposed to help me deal with this, said Donnie. The pills do work. You don't like how they make you look and feel so you don't take em. Why me? My brothers ain't like this. Neither is my sister. God picks who she wants. Everyone can't be born perfect Donnie. We all have flaws. We all fall short of the glory of God. Damn! You know the bible? Donnie asked. Yeah, I know it quite well. I helped write it. We just had a misunderstanding if you will, after a meeting of the minds about the book of Genesis and Enoch. I was always told not to question God, but it feels like my hand is forced. I've been praying since I was little and I'm still the same. The bible says you can do all things through Christ. Why ain't nothing working for me Roman? Why Peter and The Boogeyman always picking on me? I ain't did nothing to them. When you had that breakdown a few hours ago, I was able to whisper in your ear, twenty dwarfs took turns doing handstands on the carpet. I didn't want them to hurt you so that's was what I used to calm you down. Once you repeated it six hundred and sixty six times, you would become silent. So, you saying you got me out of there? Donnie asked. Why you helping me Roman? Because I feel that I could use you. You can be an asset to me. You got the looks and the savagery. It's better to reign in hell than to serve in heaven Donnie. I've been here with my nose in dinosaur's asses since the whole thing began. Every sensation and want a man was inspired to have, I nurtured that, not God. I cared about what man wanted and I never judged them. That's why I'm more popular today than I've ever been. I'm loved here on earth. The music industry, media, and sports. It's all mine. They worship me. They know of God, but they really obey with me. I'm everything. I'm a vibe. I won't lead you astray. I won't abandon you like God and your family did. Who can deny that the twentieth century is all mine Donnie? I give man everything, God sells hope. I'm in my prime Donnie. I can stop the voices right now if you follow me. I can even fix your brain for you. What say you? Are you all in? Are you ready to join my army of soldiers? If it's money you want Donnie, I have more than the law allows. All you have to do is lay down your cross and follow me. I'm all you have left. You haven't heard a peep from Peter and The Boogeyman, right? I got that under control. Are you in Donnie?

Gary G. McDonald

I, I, I don't know. What all do I have to do? We can discuss that later Donnie. I can take away the voices and make you regular right now if that's what you want. I'll tell you what you owe me later. Can you make me rich too? Donnie asked. Anything you want. Can I be famous? People will really know who I am? Yep. Can I be on tv too? Anything your heart desire Donnie. I own the earth and everything in it remember? Yeah, I remember, Donnie said nervously. Let me think about it. Give me a few days and I'll give you my answer. A few days? Roman asked. Are you kidding me? Who does that? I give you the opportunity to rid yourself of these mean ass voices, bring your family back and make you rich and you need some time to think. What the fuck Donnie? Roman shouted. You're pissing me off. This is what you wanted right? So, take it! Now I see why people always fucking with you can't get right. You ain't shit. You have the chance of a lifetime to heal yourself and become regular, and you wanna think about it. Niggas! I tell ya. Alright Donnie. This is what I'll do for you. Since I like you, and you have nobody else you can count on, I'll give you twenty four hours. That's the least I can do, since my friend God didn't help you. Twenty four hours Donnie. That's a whole day to do some thinking. I want you to really reflect on the type of life you want and deserve, from this point on. You won't hear any voices. The police won't stop you. It'll be just you by your lonesome, clearing your mind of all the negative things that you've been through. Let the hurt of that little boy trapped inside of you go. Let me in Donnie. I will protect you from the world. I'll keep you out of jail. You'll be above the law. Can you imagine having a life of a celebrity Donnie? Everything you've always dreamed of and wanted to have is within your reach. I still have my sister and my brother John. I'm not fully alone Roman. Oh really? Ok, Donnie. I was going to give you twenty four hours of silence while you make up your mind but fuck it. Think while God ignores you, and I'll let Peter and The Boogeyman torment you. Put that in your pipe and smoke it bro. You better have your mind made up by tomorrow night, no later than 10:34 pm. The clock is ticking. This is your one chance to have the freedom you wanted. Take it! Roman shouted. Bye Donnie. But before I go, I want to leave you with this. Roman 3:16. Destruction and misery are in their ways. And the way of peace, they have not known. There is no fear of God before their eyes. I'm the total package Donnie. You either do as I say and obey me, or you stay this way. Join a winning team, said Roman. Like I said, I'll think about it, Donnie replied. Ok, do you.

Roman snaps his finger loudly, and the voices return immediately. Donnie's clock was ticking. He was so immersed into his conversation with the devil, he didn't notice the drug users, prostitutes, pimps and passerby's all staring at him while he was talking to himself.

Hey man, you alright? Bro you ok? A dope fiend asked. Hey you? Hey what's good. Donnie asked. You good? Yeah, I'm Ok, said Donnie.
Handsome

Donnie why the fuck have you been ignoring us? Me and The, boogeyman feel neglected. What were you doing? How were you able to block us out? You discovered a new method of resistance huh? Peter asked. God why did you choose for me to be this way? The devil wants to make a deal with me to have a good life and I'm thinking about taking it. I have nothing else to lose. I know the Bible says, what's a man to gain the whole world but lose his soul, but I've been mentally fucked up for years. I finally have a chance at a normal life, and it sounds very tempting. Where are you? Can you help me or guide me in the right direction? Hello? God are you there? I'm depressed and suicidal. My family's gone and I'm all alone. Are you going to help me or no? Donnie shouted.

The crowd of people gathered in the park took a few steps backwards the louder Donnie's voice had gotten. It's hard to make dope fiends and killers nervous, and Donnie did just that.

God don't like you Donnie Boy. If he did, he wouldn't have made you this way. God abandoned you like your family did. We're all you have. Fuck you Peter. Aye, there's my boy. There's that fire mouth. You should go run out in front of a car and let everybody watch your brains get splattered all over the road. Boo! Donnie shouts. God if you don't stop them, I swear I'm going to take a handful of pills. I can silence them forever if you don't. I know you don't want us destroying you creations but I'm all out of options, plus you won't answer. Asking God to fix your stupid ass is like asking him to make you white. It's impossible. Won't happen, said Peter. Fuck you. Twenty dwarfs took turns doing handstands on the carpet. Twenty dwarfs took turns doing handstands on the carpet. Twenty dwarfs took turns doing handstands on the carpet. Twenty dwarfs took turns doing handstands on the carpet. Uh Oh, there he goes down the rabbit hole. Keep going Donnie, you're almost there. Snap out of it Donnie, Roman shouts. I'm depressed and sad like you. We should sit in the corner and cry. Stop yelling at him, Peter and the Boogeyman. You know he's not strong enough to block us out. Give him a break. God still has protection over him and his soul. You have 23 hours and 15 minutes Donnie, Roman whispered. Stop it guys. Just let him be. You can stop this at anytime Donnie, Roman whispers. I'm nothing but a worthless basket case with no options. That's the spirit. Keep that same energy Donnie. You're almost there. A little bit more. Ain't nothing here for me. I love it Donnie. You're on a roll. Stop prolonging this bro. Slit your wrist. Go up the canal and not across you chicken. You'll be on the other side in no time. Then you'll be able to tell us if Heaven or Hell is real, says Peter. I still think we should go out and kill a few white people, said The Boogeyman. They'll never suspect us. Most serial killers are white, shit, probably all of them are. But they'll never look your way Donkey. What you say? Are you with it?

Gary G. McDonald

NO! I'm not turning into no damn serial killer. You do it, Donnie shouts. We can't do anything with out you. You're the key to starting a panic around here. Chicago has enough black on black crime to deal with, let's do some white people shit. I promise we won't kill any of our people, The Boogeyman said convincingly. I ain't killing nobody. I have the chance to be famous and rich. I have the chance to be on tv. If I listen to yall, like I did all the other times, I'll miss out on this once in a lifetime opportunity, Donnie said calmly. My son and daughter is all I have from my lineage. I have to set good examples for them and create generational wealth for them too. I hope they don't inherit this dreadful disease. Why would an all, powerful deity, create an imperfect human being? Don't ask me shit. Ask God? Fuck you Peter! My name binit and I ain't in it. Do your own due diligence. If I were you, I'd give God a piece of my mind though. Or you could do us all a favor and just kill yourself. You're a waste of fresh air.

Donnie reaches in the bottom of his shoe and removes the sole. Underneath was a straight razor that he used to slice his arm up in the park. Witnesses were stunned and took off their shirts to help wrap the wounds. The ambulance was called, but by then, Donnie walked off to a payphone. He called his brother John and told him he needed somewhere to stay and that he was homeless. John was happy to hear from his brother and put Donnie on hold and called Shante 3-way. Being his brother's keeper over the years came with a lot of responsibilities, fights and headaches, but John never gave up hope. And now that they were grown, he really felt the need to keep him closer. Growing up, John often feared that the streets or prison life would kill Donnie, if he didn't kill them first. People living with mental illnesses are easy targets because they stand out. They indirectly make themselves known to people, with little to no understanding about the disease. In return, they're beaten, harmed, spit on, and disrespected in such dehumanizing ways.

Hey Shante. Hey John. Everything ok with you in New York? Shante asked. Yeah, everything's great so far. It's not me I'm calling about, it's Donnie. What's wrong with Donnie? Is he alright? Kind of sort of, John replied. Could your brother stay with you for a few weeks until he moves up here with me in New York? Shante was reluctant on letting her brother come to stay with her because she had young kids in the house. Donnie was unpredictable, especially growing up. She's always lived in fear around him lowkey but never said anything because he was family. Shante agreed to let him stay for two weeks and not a minute more. Donnie spoke with his landlord that same evening to retrieve his things the next morning. Donnie promised to abide by his siter's rules and agreed to her terms and conditions. The clock was still ticking for Donnie's deal with the devil as he headed towards Tay's house.

Handsome
Chapter 16

What You Not Gone Do

By winter, Donnie was all settled in at his sister's place, with her and his nieces and nephews. He was back to work at his old job at Gold Bloom Baking and things were going well for him. Sheila had spread a rumor at work that Donnie flipped out on her during a date. The employees were constantly whispering and pointing their fingers at Donnie during breaks. He tried to ignore the rumors and voices in his head, but to no avail. This was Donnie's second write up for loud talking and misconduct. His baking skills spoke for him. Management have always had difficult employees to deal with, but not someone that could bake as good as Donnie. They didn't want to lose him, so they gave him a promotion. He was ecstatic about his new position. Word got out that they were about to have a new supervisor. Sheila and some of the people that were pointing fingers weren't to thrilled about Donnie being their boss. A few of them threatened to quit, stating that they weren't going to take orders from a crazy person, and they feared for their lives. Management held a meeting with the staff and ensured them that if there was a problem, they would take the blame. And that if anyone was hurt due to his negligence, they'll be fully compensated.

Deep down inside Donnie felt betrayed by Sheila and was upset that she went back to work talking shit about him and their date. But, was happy at the same time that his skills weren't going unnoticed by management. He was embarrassed by the finger pointing and neglected to ask for a ride home, so he walked instead. After arriving home some forty minutes later, all sweaty and tired, Donnie walked into the house and slammed the door.

Who slamming doors in my motherfucking house? Shante asked in a rage. My bad sis. Yo bad? Yo bad? You damn right it's yo bad. What you not gone do is be coming up in here all big and bad slamming my damn door. I told you before you got here to respect my house. It was just a matter of time before you showed your ass. Sis, I ain't do nothing but slam the door. I ain't try to, it just sort of happened. I wasn't thinking. I apologize sis. That's your damn problem now, you never think. You just do, Shante shouted. Always about Donnie and what Donnie want. I put up with enough of your shit growing up, I don't need it in my adult life too around my kids. C'mon now sis, you yelling at me like I'm your child or something. Or one of those lame ass baby daddies of yours. Boy, what you not gone do is be raising your voice in my house. Yo the one wrong, and you slamming doors like you own this bitch. Yeah you help me pay a bill or two, and I appreciate it. But don't be bringing that negative shit from out there in my positive space. Your day was probably bad, mine was good. You see how happy I look? Shante asked with an attitude.

Gary G. McDonald

Why you always tripping on me sis? I thought you loved me. I ain't never did nothing to you. All you need is a good man in your life Tay, you won't be so uptight. You need a chump to occupy your time and let you push him around. I hope one of these niggas take that stick out of your ass and put a smile on your tight ass face. Tight ass? A stick in my ass? Boy, I know damn well you done last your rabbit ass mind. Trying me in my house. Let me shut up. I almost went there with you Donnie. This was a favor for John. Gone ahead about your business before I say something I'll regret. Don't bite your tongue now sis. Speak yo mind. You ain't never like me anyways. You always been mean to me. You laughed and played with everybody but me. That shit used t hurt my feelings Tay. Like you said it was a favor for John, other than that you wouldn't give a shit if I lived or died. Donnie, what you not gone is be telling me how the fuck I feel. Your disrespectful ass came in here slamming doors and I wasn't supposed to say nothing about it. You got life twisted baby brother. Despite of what you think, I do love you. I just do it from a distance and not close up like everyone else. That's how I choose to deal with you, Tay yelled. This my house. I could talk how the fuck I want. If you don't like it, you can leave. I can't wat until you move with John, I'll be able to have my house back and my boys can sleep in their own rooms again. Yeah yeah. And all of this I thought I was the only one crazy. You're a bug too Tay. That's why ain't no men around. You keep running them away with that big mouth of yours. Boy, your big head ass got some fucking nerves. You don't know what goes on in my house. Listen, I ain't trying to go back and forth with you. Blood don't make us family huh sis. Donnie, I'm gone excuse the dumb shit you saying right now because your elevator don't go all the way up. I'll spare you the insults. Whatever Tay. If I had a car I would've been gone. Boy, ain't nobody stopping you. That's why I'm saving money now sis. I just need two more weeks and I'm out of your hair for good. Thanks for giving me a place to stay Tay. Sorry again for slamming your door. Don't be trying to talk all nice now. Keep that same energy you had earlier, Tay said as she walked behind him. I ain't fixing fight you sis. Boy bye. That's what I thought.

Donnie walks into his room and purposely slams the door. This time the door comes off the hinges. Shante rushes into the room and starts to punch on her much bigger brother. She violently threw punches at Donnie as if he was someone on the streets. Shante had just as much built up anger inside of her and it had to be released. Donnie was the only person around for her to take out her frustrations.

Why you hitting me sis? Girl you bat shit crazy. And you sitting here berating me but look at you. Look at the pot calling the kettle black, said Shante. Ain't that some shit. These two weeks better hurry up and come. I don't know how much more of this I can take. You gone be done had me on the tonight's news messing with you.
Handsome

Let me leave you alone before you really go banana split in here, Shante said jokingly. Ma will flip over in her grave if she heard how you talked to me today, said Donnie. She would be appalled at your behavior. This nigga done learned some new words in prison, trying to use that shit on me. Boy bye. What you not gone do is keep trying to bring mama into this. Stand on your own too feet for a change. She don't wanna hear about your grown ass man problems. And you talking about moving to New York, the police just as racist up there than they are here. That big ass mouth will surely get you in trouble. You already been to prison a bunch of times, you need to go up there and chill the fuck out before your ass end up dead. Ain't nothing gonna happen to me, I'm Donnie P. Boy, you ain't shit. You or Donnie P. Clean up this junkie ass room. Yes mother. Right away mother, Donnie said facetiously. If you don't like it Donnie, there's the door. Don't let the door "hitcha" where the good lord "splitcha". You'll be sad when I move. You ain't got nobody else trying to be around your annoying ass. That's why you picking on me. You're bored and backed up. You're my sister, you shouldn't be treating me this way. I ain't never treat you like this. I was always nice to you, Donnie said calmly. I'm just be gone be real with you brother. You probably don't remember half the shit you do when you're off your meds or under the influence of drugs or alcohol, so I'll tell you. I'll give you a trip down memory lane and hopefully this does something to refresh your thoughts. I'll go back to when I was about seven. You took the heads off of all of my baby dolls and buried them in the backyard. Or the one time I caught you standing over me in your sleep holding a butcher knife. Or the time you set my entire school project on fire. The papers and the actual project. Shall I continue Donnie? So, excuse me if I don't give you the brother of the year award. This ain't what you want Donnie. You stay in your lane and I'll stay in mine. Capisce? Shante asked. Hurry up and get your funds together so that you could move with your brother. He's gonna be happy to see you. People with illnesses like you Donnie don't comprehend things like the rest of us. That's why I try not to be so hard on you, but you have my hands tied behind my back sometimes. Then I'm forced to be this mean sister. You won't let a motherfucker be nice to you. It's ok though sis, we're all designed differently. I get it. You started with me Tay, I ain't do nothing but slam the door. You act like the world ending. Slamming the door and making it come off the hinges is a big deal. Housing comes by and do walk through's. They're gonna ask me what happened to the door. It'll be on me to fix it and the take incident reports. Just fix the damn door, expeditiously please. Thank you and bye. Whatever, Donnie mumbled. That's all she d is talk shit. Somebody need o put some dick in her life and in her mouth. Mean ass! I can't stand her spiteful lonely ass. A few more dollars and I'm out of here. Fuck Tay! She'll miss me when I'm gone. She always trying to embarrass somebody. Big loudmouth, ass. I can't stand her. Ugh. What you not gone do Donnie is keep mumbling under your breath in my house like some little ass boy. Fix your life Donnie and my damn door.
Gary G. McDonald

Chapter 17

Naked and Afraid

A week later, during a late night argument with his sister Shante, Donnie said some things he shouldn't have. He was put out in the cold Chicago weather with his belongings with nowhere to go. Shante had enough of his bad attitude towards her and his erratic behavior. She knew that letting Donnie come to live with her was suspect from the start, but that was her brother. Donnie had no one to turn too and wore out his welcome everywhere except for with John. By then he'd saved up enough money to buy him a car but decided to hold on to it for a one way ticket, and a fresh start in New York. Donnie only needed another three days and he would've been out of Chicago anyways. The first night out of Shante's house, he took his things and tried to sleep on a park bench. That wasn't going to work because of his trust issues and mental illnesses. Fiends were all over the park. Some were there to get high, and others were there looking for a place to crash. At night the parks were always full of weirdos and people having sex in wide open, not to mention a plethora of used and exposed needles laying around. The smell of sex and drugs polluted the air along with Covid- 19. But nobody seemed to care. The world was moving in slow motion for Donnie. Growing up, because of Donnie's mental illnesses, he was always cautious, and his head was always on a swivel. This was his second time in life where he actually had to sleep outside with no other alternatives. His mother was always there for him to lean on when things got rough, and now that she was gone it was more harder for him to focus. Before sunup, Donnie went into the shitty park bathroom to splash some water on his face, brush his teeth and to take a bird bath. A bird bath is when you get water from an unknown or reliable source to wash off quickly. Mainly your hot spots. Which are your under arms and private areas. After getting so fresh and so clean, Donnie walked over to the neighborhood bodega.

Hi, good morning Sir. Can I have a black and mild please? Donnie asked. Ok my friend, that'll be $1.50, said the Arabic clerk. Here you go. Thank you. Have a nice day, said Donnie. I go to find somewhere to stay for the night. I'll get a motel. I have more than enough for two nights. Man, stop being a pussy, The Boogeyman shouted. Let's break in a motherfuckers house. Tie them up and chill there for a few days. You could save your money. We could kill them too if you'd like. I'm already out here in the cold with nowhere to go and now you're aggravating the shit out of me. Leave me the fuck alone. Donnie shouted. Why would I do that Donnie Boy? I told you before, we're friends to the end like Chucky. I'll never leave you. We're joined at the hip. The brain too, now that I think about it. I am you Donnie, and you're me. I thought you weren't supposed to come back. He tricked me. Who Donnie?
        Handsome

Never mind. It doesn't matter. All lives matter Donnie. Fuck you Peter! Black Lives Matter. Period. Fuck you mean all lives? They killing our people every day. Where's your sympathy for them. I wish I could cut you out of my brain. You be saying a lot of stupid shit. I'm you Donnie, you don't make since 90 percent of the time. You ain't shit Peter. That's all you do is talk shit. Blah blah blah. Fuck all of that you're talking about. Are we sleeping outside or you going to kill for us? The clocks ticking. What's it going to be? It's cold as fuck out here nigga. Make up your mind. If not make up with your sister and let's get some shelter. He's right Donnie. Let's scare the shit out of a few people. Make them piss their pants. Or dresses, The Boogeyman says jokingly. The time is now, to get even with all of those that bullied you and made you feel worthless. Do something about it. Do it! Do it! The voices collectively shouted. We need to get on some and celebrate before running off to New York, said The Boogeyman. Let's get really high and by the time we get to New York, we'll be super lit. We could sit back and relax on the train in peace. Donnie booked a cabin We should play who done it and strangle some passengers on the train, said The Boogeyman. I swear Donnie, sometimes you're no fun. You love to sit around and sulk. You like feeling sorry for yourself. Shut your pie hole, Donnie shouts. I made a deal for you to disappear and someone reneged on it. What deal? I already told you that I'm an unstoppable force. Ain't no getting rid of me. You're delusional Donnie. That's your new name from here on out, Delusional Donnie. I fucking hate it here. Go and find someone else to torture and torment. Twenty dwarfs took turns doing handstands on the carpet. Twenty dwarfs took turns doing handstands on the carpet. Twenty dwarfs took turns doing handstands on the carpet, Donnie said repeatedly. There you go Delusional Donnie, go down that rabbit hole of yours. I'm Peter Cottontail, I'm coming with you. Create another voice why don't ya. You take us everywhere you go anyways, like an American Express card. You never leave home without us. Donnie, can you hear me? Donnie. Hello Donnie. Yeah, I can hear you, Donnie replied. Who are you? I'm from the future. You can't get on that train and go to New York tomorrow. It's imperative that you stay. The police are going to kill you in Rochester. Tell your brother John you changed your mind. But whatever you do, you can not come to New York. This ain't a joke. I'm in the year 2034. My name is Commander George Floyd. I'm a leader in the resistance. You're supposed to do a speech here in my time and you were assassinated. You are an expert on the topic of mental health and your life does matter as well as black ones. Stay there in Chicago for another day or two until this all blows over. Why should I believe you? Donnie asked. I don't know how I can make you believe me, but I do know this. If you get on that train, you're a dead man. My brother wants me to move out there, I can't disappoint him. If you get on that train, you die. There's nothing more I can say. My time here has run out. We need you in the future Donnie. Whatever you do, don't go to Rochester. This is Commander Floyd of the Resistance, and I'm out. Peace.
                Gary G. McDonald

Hey John. What's good? I heard you fucked up and got put out of your sisters, with only three days left. Damn Donnie. You sure you're ok to come up here? John asked worriedly. It wasn't my fault. Shante was riding me since I got there for slamming a door one day. I had a bad day at work and slammed it by accident. I forgot where I was and who I was dealing with. She never let up John. She was constantly at me. I told her she needed some dick to calm her down, and that's what sent her over the edge. She was always at a point of no return. Then she told me shit I did when we were little that made her hate me even more. I could've been the nicest person that day, and she still would've found a reason to be upset. When you living under someone else's roof, those are some of the things you go through. That's why you have to get your own place Donnie. I'm going to get a room here for a couple of nights at this motel, and I'll be up your way. That shit with Tay wasn't my fault big bro. It's always someone else's fault Donnie. You can't keep placing the blame on other people. You gotta take responsibility for your actions. Now you coming down on me too John. Nah Donnie, I'm just saying, your behavior gets you into a lot of trouble, mainly when you don't take your meds. I know I know. I'm trying to do better bro. I'm not perfect. It's a struggle everyday living with this shit. Just when I think I'm doing good, I'm not. It's a fucking rollercoaster John. I'm not sure if I'm strong enough mentally to handle this any longer. This guy George Floyd, from the future told me not to come there. He said the police gone kill me John. I don't want to die big bro. I just want to come up there and live with you. We've always been the closest and I believe you gone watch out for me. But I'm scared. Who is George Floyd? He was talking to me in my head. He said he was from the future and my life had meaning. He said I was a mental health specialist and I'm supposed to do a speech in the year 2034. Do you hear how you sound Donnie? Them people gone lock yo ass up before you get here. Have you taken your meds today? Yes, I have Donnie replied with an attitude. I wish everybody would stop asking me that. Just do me a favor little brother and stay out of trouble for the next few days. The police killing unarmed black men and women around the country, even kids. You have to be safe and stay indoors. No walking around or any sightseeing. Stay out of them people face and make it here in one piece. Can you do that Donnie? Make it here in one piece? I can do that John. I'll keep my nose clean. You can't afford anymore attention that could send you back to prison. I hear you John. I promise I'll stay in the room and out of the way. You have children to live for Donnie. It's not just you anymore. You have two lives that want their father in their lives. Don't let them down. Be there for them like mama was for us. I think I did something stupid, but I don't know yet. I gotta see how it plays out. It ain't nothing that could me to jail, I'm just saying. I'll let you know how it goes. What the hell you talking about Donnie? I made a deal with the devil to stop these voices and to make me rich. You what? Boy go take your meds. You really tripping now. A deal with the devil, John says jokingly. I did. I'm about to be rich.
                                         Handsome

Ok bro. You're about to be famous. I get it. I'm for real. The devil said he's going to stop the voices and make me rich. Ha ha ha , John laughs. Are you still hearing voices? Yeah. There's your answer. You're making excuse on why not to come. The devil and people from the future and shit. Listen to yourself Donnie. You need help. I'm here trying to provide that, along with a safe haven for you. It's all about what you want out of life little brother. I know John, I was just saying that trouble can find me anywhere. You ever heard of a dude named Eric Garner that died up there in 2014? No. Who is that? John asked. A black guy, hanging out selling cd's in front of a bodega. Police came up and choked him out. They killed the dude for no reason. The officers were later fired but acquitted on the charges. That's why I've been hesitating John. It's scary in New York too. I could die anywhere. Understandable Donnie. I get it. I just can't afford to lose you too. We're all we got Donnie. Ain't nobody else here to help you. Be safe little brother. See you in a few days, I got to get dressed for work. Love you Donnie. Everything's going to be ok. You just make it here safe. Love you too John.

The brothers hang up the phone and continue going about their day. Donnie checked into a motel for the night and was going to be on the first train smoking. After settling in, Peter convinced Donnie to get high on PCP before the twenty one hour ride so that he could relax. PCP is a powerful street drug that causes hallucinations and distorts a persons perception of reality. Donnie went out that night and found just what he was looking for. He got back to his room and proceeded to get high. Peter rant and raves throughout the night and doesn't allow Donnie to get any sleep. Later that evening around 10 pm, Donnie's sister Shante calls his cell phone and tells him that their nephew committed suicide. Their brother Bryan's son battled with depression. He and Donnie were pretty close and often joked about their mental illnesses. Now, he was feeling like his world was ending. Everyone he knew was dead except for John and Shante. Someone was always dying before their time in Donnie's life. The Devil was trying to get his attention for the second time as he continued to get high on PCP. The world was going up in flames in Donnie's mind. The more he smoked, the more paranoid and irrational he had gotten. He paced back and forth on the dampened smelling carpet, as he repeatedly peeked out of his room window. Donnie stayed up all night tweaking. He was team, no sleep. His body was tired and his mental stability as at an all time low. As he continued to get high, Donnie's heart stopped. He was looking up at the ceiling with his eyes wide open. He grabs his heart and starts praying to God.

Hey Donnie. Remember me? It's Roman. Bring your life to me and I'll make it better. How long will I live? Donnie asked. Eternal life and forever, says Roman. Will I be the same handsome Donnie? You'll have the life that you've always dreamed of. Just relax your soul and let me take control. Close your eyes Donnie. My eyes are closed.
     Gary G. McDonald

The next morning before boarding the train, Donnie buys a $20 scratch off and wins the Chicago's Grand Prize of $10 million dollars. His mental illnesses doesn't allow him to get excited. It was just another day for him. He folds his winning ticket and puts it in his back pocket. Roman boast about his powers and reassures Donnie that his move to New York was in his best interest and that he'll never leave his side. There was one stipulation though. He couldn't tell a soul about the deal he made with the devil, and if he did, there would be dire consequences. Their deal would be off. Null and void. Donnie agrees to his terms and conditions.

Do you have your boarding pass Sir? The Conductor asked. Is everything ok? You're sweating really bad. It's a virus out there killing people, says the Conductor. No, I'm ok. I was running so that I didn't miss my ride. I'll get some paper towels and wipe my face once I get to the restroom. Alright Sir. Watch your step. Thank you, Sir. Hi ma'am. Where's your restroom? In the next car over, to the right, said the attendant. Ok thanks ma'am.

Donnie rushes into the restroom and splashes water on his face. The PCP had him all jacked up from the night before. On top of that, he failed to take his medications as prescribed for the last two days. His reality wasn't ours. In his world, everyone was gone with the exception of his brother. He was all over the place and so were his eyes. He was mentally unstable and physically unable to make the arduous journey from Illinois to New York. Shortly after the train pulls off from the station, Donnie's erratic behavior kicks into overdrive. Passengers weren't sure of what to make of the handsome black guy talking to himself. Several passengers stopped to ask Donnie if he was ok, but he doesn't respond. He kept repeating, twenty dwarfs took turns doing handstands on the carpet for several miles. The authorities were alerted of Donnie's behavior. After a brief conversation with the conductor, it was determined by the authorities that Donnie was perhaps under the influence of drugs. Nobody questioned the possibility of him having a nervous breakdown or him suffering from mental illnesses, they automatically assumed drugs from the jump. Donnie was asked to get his things as he was politely removed from the train, for the safety of everyone on board. He was stranded in Ohio with no other way of getting to New York. Donnie knew that John would be upset with him for getting high and being put off the train, so he decided to hitchhike. That was the only way of making it there on time. There was 18 hours remaining before he was due to arrive at Union Station. After two hours of standing near the interstate with his thumb out, a female pulls over and asked where he was going. Donnie tells the young lady that he was headed to New York. She tells him to get in and that it was his lucky day because that's where she was going.

Handsome

Donnie struck up a good conversation with the young lady to break the ice. The Boogeyman was suggesting that he choke the driver and steal her car. Donnie kept his composure and did his best to ignore him. The ride was easy going and there was no erratic behavior the entire ride. They talked for hours about all sorts of things, even doing a little flirting.

Seventeen hours and forty two minutes later, the pair had pulled into Union Station with time to spare. Donnie thanks the beautiful driver and hands her the $10 million dollar scratch off not knowing how much he'd really won. It's not much, he tells her, and thanks the young lady again. Donnie calls his brother and lets him know that he arrived earlier than expected and to come pick him up. John got into his vehicle and didn't waste any time on going to get his little brother.

I'm glad you came John. You? I'm excited as hell little brother. You're finally here and away from those bad influences. Do you know how scared I was for you out in Chicago? It seems like every day I would turn on the news, Chicago was on there. I'm talking about nothing but murders. Children out there being killed. I hoped and prayed that I wouldn't get a phone call of you being shot and killed by those gang bangers or the police. I'm just happy you're here. You have no idea bro, said John. I'm good bro. I'm in one piece like you said to come in big brother. I'm happy to be here too. I'm gone make the best of this. I promise. I'm gonna find me a job and get my own place like you John. Thanks again for letting me live with you. Shante was tripping. Did she call you too and tell you about Bryan's son? Yeah, she called and told me. It's sad how he took his own life, said John. Man, I thought about it and tried killing myself so much throughout the years, I lost track. Living with schizophrenia, we see differently and feel differently from everyone else John. My doctor recently put me on Caplyta. It's a new medicine they wanted me to try out. Hopefully it helps me. This change to New York is what I needed brother. I was getting tired of the same old same old. A lot of people fear change. The unknown scares people John. I know it does, John replied. I had to get out of there. After nephew died that was my que to leave Chicago and never look back. Shit was piling up on me back in Chicago. People at work was on me, Tay was tripping, and my girl left me. My life was all fucked up there. You saved my John. I hope I can come and do a 360 turn around. I also want to stop drinking and getting high. I think that's what causes me to have a lot of problems. I'm going to monitor my behavior on this new drug Caplyta, without PCP and alcohol in my life. It's a start brother. One day at a time. Rome wasn't built in a day you know. Things like that takes time, it's not an overnight fix. I'm going to be here to help see you through it all Donnie. I'm your number one fan. Thanks, big brother. Thanks for loving me and always having my back like you promised since we were kids. You're welcome Donnie. That's what brothers are for.

Gary G. McDonald

I promised mama that I'll always be my brother's keeper and I have. She's proud of you for that John. Everybody gave up on me except for you. You don't know how much I cherish that. You've been consistent for over thirty something years straight on having my back. That's mind blowing big brother. It was apart of my job. You needed this change of scenery Donnie. It'll help you become more mentally stable. I hope so bro. You want to play movie trivia John? C'mon let's go little brother. Ok ok. I never liked you anyways, you pretty motherfucker. What movie that's from John? Too easy. Wrong. No, I was saying the question was too easy. The answer is New Jack City, said John. Aw man. Ok ok. I got another one, says Donnie. I don't get involved with anyone I can't walk out on in sixty seconds or less if I feel the heat coming around the corner? Heat, John says quickly. With Robert Deniro and Al Pacino. Damn you are good. I'm a movie buff Donnie. I've seen and heard it all before. That's a classic movie. You're better than me at this game. You better know it, said John. The opening was gangster as hell too. But that bank shootout was everything though. It really was. One of the best that I've ever seen, Donnie says with excitement. It be so much going on in my head. I can't seem to tune in on things that are important. This mental illness a motherfucker. People look at me weird and treat me differently than they treat everyone else. Nobody gives me a chance to show them anything other than my bad side. I try my hardest not to be this way, but I can't help it. I can't keep a relationship because it. Do you have a girlfriend John? No, I have a wife now. A wife When did you get married? I got married last year. We met at church one day and went out for dinner a few times and the rest is history. We've been together since. You don't remember I invited you to come be in the wedding? John asked. Nah. You know what? I do remember that. I think I was in jail around that time. Yea you went to jail the week after I invited you. My bad big bro. Everybody's dead. We're all alone John. You know that? We're not alone Donnie. It's all in your head. Don't focus on the past, think about the future. Think about the here and now. Think about the opportunities you have here in New York. It's a big ass city Donnie. You could be anything you'd like. Sky's the limit. I know John. I go to take it all in. Once I get settled, maybe I'll be able to think differently. I'm afraid though. That dude from the future told me not to come out here. He said the police was going to shoot me. There you go. I thought I just told you to think positively. Talking about someone in your head from the future isn't helping the situation Donnie. Focus brother, focus. No more talk about the people in your head. Keep that stuff to yourself. Don't share that information with people. Your problems will follow you here to New York if you do. Alright John. No more talking about the people in my head. I got it. You miss mama them? Yep. All the time. When I say my prayers, I say hi to them. I also ask God to watch over you too. Thanks John. I appreciate it.

Handsome

No problem little brother. You miss Chicago John? Nope. I do. I miss it a lot. I feel home sick. I've never been this far from home before. That's not your home anymore, this is. Leave all of your worries and troubles behind you. This your chance to have a fresh start where nobody knows you. I understand John. Making your way in the world today, takes everything you got. Taking a break from all of my worries, would surely help a lot. Wouldn't you like to get away? But sometimes you want to go where everybody knows your name. People are always glad you came. You want to be where you can see, troubles are all the same. You to go where everybody knows your name John. Donnie, did you just use the song to Cheers to say that? John asked jokingly. Oh, that's where that came from? My bad. It was in my head.

They started laughing as they continued down the freeway. Donnie looked around in amazement at the tall buildings that he only saw on tv. He starts to sweat profusely and began repeating twenty dwarfs took turns doing handstands on the carpet.

Donnie are you ok? Donnie. What the fuck yo? Donnie. Answer me bro. Twenty dwarfs took turns doing handstands on the carpet. Twenty dwarfs took turns doing handstands on the carpet. Twenty dwarfs took turns doing handstands on the carpet. Donnie chill out, please. C'mon little brother, chill out. You're not acting like you took your meds. We're almost to my place.

John takes out his phone and calls his wife to alert her of his brother's erratic behavior. She gets his room prepared and await their arrival.

We're almost there Donnie, just sit tight bro. C'mon light, change. Almost there Donnie, hold on. Twenty dwarfs took turns doing handstands on the carpet. I know that movie Donnie, it's Bugsy. God watch over my little brother. He means well. Wrap your shield of protection around him God. Help him Lord God. Please. He needs you more than anything. Damn Donnie, how you get all the way to New York and do this now. You got to be kidding me. C'mon Donnie, snap out of it. Twenty dwarfs took turns doing handstands on the carpet. Twenty dwarfs took turns doing handstands on the carpet. I'm still not situated like I would like to be, and I was bringing you out here for you to have a better life than what you had in Chicago. We're here Donnie. Unfasten your seat belt. C'mon bro I got you. I ain't going to let anything happen to you. C'mon Donnie. You're sweating bad bro. Did you take drugs before coming here? Donnie. You on drugs bro? I'm thirsty John. Can I have some water please. I'm thirsty bro. I need some water. Please. C'mon, watch your step. I got you. Babe, come here and help me. There you go Donnie. One step at a time. I got you Donnie. C'mon. Easy does it.

Gary G. McDonald

Stay right here Donnie while I get you luggage. Ok John. Twenty dwarfs took turns doing handstands on the carpet. Shh. Chill out bro. We can't have that around here. You hear that John? No brother. Stay there. I'm coming. Let me get you some water.

John runs into the kitchen to get his brother a bottle of water and urges him to drink all of it to cool off. Donnie paced back and forth as he took the bottle of water to the head. John runs and gets him another bottle of water at Donnie's request. John was really worried for his brother and was unsure if he was on drugs or off of his meds. John hugs his brother and tells him that everything was going to be ok. He continues on trying to keep his brother calm, but to no avail. As John tries walks his brother to the basement where he would be staying, Donnie goes against the grain and tells his brother about Roman.

Roman is a crazy little boy that lives inside of me. He says all of the things I don't want to say, and he fights my battles. He was born the other day and created from rage. He's able to keep the other voices quiet. He's the devil, but he uses the name Roman. I asked him and the others to leave, but he won't go. He says he owns me and my soul John. Can you believe it?

Before John could utter a word, Donnie jumps headfirst down the stairs into the basement. His wife immediately calls 911, stating that her brother in law suffering from mental illnesses had went headfirst down a flight of stairs. The operator said that an ambulance was in route and should be there shortly. Paramedics arrive shortly after and take Donnie to Strong Memorial Hospital to be evaluated. John was visibly upset about his brothers condition and what had transpired. He was confused about how this could be happening to his brother the first day in New York. Later that evening Donnie was seen by several nurses and released from the hospital at around 11 pm. Both nurses that looked after Donnie had come to the same conclusion. Donnie was given a ride from the hospital by one of the caretakers and returned home. Things were calm and Donnie ate him a hefty dinner plate and went to lay down in his new room. John thought the medications and the visit to the hospital was all that he needed, until Donnie asked for a cigarette and took off running barefoot down the street. Not to mention it was freezing and raining by this time. He ran down the street as if someone was chasing after him. John called police out to his residence for the second time in less than 24 hours for his mentally ill brother. He also cautioned the police not to hurt his brother because he was harmless. Reports came in about 3 am. It was March 30th 2020 that a man was seen naked, bleeding and disoriented walking in the middle of the road. Police arrive on the seen and encounter Donnie with no clothes on, casually walking in the rain.

Handsome

Sir. Are you ok? Sir, where are you clothes? The officer asked. Are you ok? Your brother said that you needed help. That's what we're here for. Man fuck you pig. I don't need your help. Leave me the fuck alone. I ain't bothering yall. You can't be wandering the streets naked Sir, says the officer. Fuck you. Leave me alone. Yall gone kill me like the man from the future said? Yall hate black people. I don't like yall either. Fuck you crackas. Nobody likes you. You don't like you. Twenty dwarfs took turns doing handstands on the carpet officer. Come walk towards us. Show me your hands. Hands up Sir. Now place them on your head, the officer commands. Fuck you pig. Sir, hands on your head.

Donnie complies with the officers request. They placed his hands behind his back and then cuffed him. Donnie's erratic behavior continued as he spit and talked shit to officers. Donnie was slammed to the pavement and his face was covered with a spit hood. There was some information circulating about the Corona Virus and police weren't taking any chances. High on PCP and full of life, Donnie continues insulting the officers and goes on a tirade.

Yall ain't shit. Yall hate black people. Yall just mad we could stay out in the sun longer than yall can. We were the first people on the planet, not yall. That's why the police always mad. I fucked your wife officer. I put all 9f this dick in her life. No didn't. Yes, I did. My whole family dead. The, man from the future said yall was going to kill me once I got to New York. I guess this what he was talking about. So, I'm about to die? I don't want to die pig. I'm sorry. I'll be good. I just wanna go back home to my brother. I should've listened to George Floyd and stayed my ass in Chicago. This some bullshit. I just got here officer. I just got here today and yall finna kill me. This shit ain't right. I sold my soul anyways. I'm gone resurrect soon. Fuck you cracka. Kiss my ass. You ain't shit and neither are you officer.

The officers get tired of Donnie's mouth and pins him to the ground by his neck. He begged and begged for his life as officers used more force to subdue him.

C'mon officer I'm sorry. I just got here. Please stop choking me. I can't breathe Sir. Please officer. I can't breathe. God help me please. Shut up nigger, God can't do a thing for you right now. Your black ass going to meet the devil. Fuck you cracka. No, fuck you nigger. This going to be your last day on this earth. Your life ain't worth shit. Niggers always screaming black lives matter. Blue lives matter motherfucker. That's the only color besides green that matter. Fuck a black life, a yellow one and red too for that matter. Fuck em all.

Donnie becomes silent and stops moving. Just like the assassination of George Floyd, he also takes his last breath.
      Gary G. McDonald

Police tried rolling Donnie over onto his side after he notices vomit and blood coming from his mouth and nose. It was too late for Donnie. The hands of time couldn't be reversed. The handsome forty one year old father, brother, uncle, baker and motivational speaker for the future resistance was dead. John called the police to go check on his brother, but not kill him. How could things have gone from bad to tragic in less than 24 hours he wondered. He was given the run around for months until he hired a lawyer to look into the disappearance of his brother. Donnie was listed as a John Doe in the City's morgue, while police plotted and planned to get rid of the incriminating video tape of the interaction between him and the police that dreadful morning. The higher up continued to hide the footage from the public. There were riots and protest following a news press conference. Donnie's brother John said publicly, that never in a million years that I would move my brother out to New York, and he ends up dead the same day.

My brother came out here to change his life and escape the gun violence that plague the streets of Chicago. He just got here to New York and yall took his life from him just like that. I'm going to get justice for Donnie, so help me God. I ain't going to rest until we get some answers. He has kids that want answers about their father's death.

The family has filed a wrongful death lawsuit against the Rochester Police Department. The officers later went before a grand jury, and nobody was indicted on any charges. The medical examiner ruled that it was cardiac arrest caused by the drug PCP, and not the spit hood or him being pinned down as the cause of death. The tragic encounter has opened the floor for discussions about the topic on mental health and how those cases are handled moving forward. Several states have implemented a crisis team be sent out instead of the police if a person is suffering from a breakdown or has mental illnesses. Donnie's life had purpose, but the people he encountered throughout his childhood and adult life didn't allow him to shine because of his mental illnesses. Once a person finds out that your mentally ill, they tend to fall back or feed you with a long handled spoon. You become a target of constant bullying, insults, and assaults. Donnie's life was full of disappointments. Death was always around the corner, taking his family members one by one. He is survived by his brother John, his sister Shante and his two kids.

Handsome

Conclusion

Mental illness is prevalent world-wide and is being widely recognized among communities of color. Unfortunately, the assistance needed to cope with this illness is not sought after or the resources aren't readily accessible to those that require it. Rather it be as a result of the lack of belief in therapy or the lack of knowledge regarding resources, our communities of color are suffering tremendously from mental illnesses. More often than not, when a person of color experiences a mental breakdown, it is not viewed as such. Their behaviors are often viewed as arrestable offenses, rather than having them Baker Acted or hospitalized to undergo an evaluation. Police are quick to make fun of the mentally disabled, the mentally ill and people of color, then it ends in tragedy. This doesn't happen in all cases, but it shouldn't happen at all. It's bad enough we're looked at as less than a human in the U.S Constitution, and they go out of their way daily to remind us of it. I would like to give a special thanks to Chalamagne Tha God, Brittney Spears, Antonio Brown, Lisa Nicole Carson, Janet Jackson, Kanye West, Little Wayne, 21 Savage, Jennifer Lewis, Jada Pinkett-Smith, Dr Tasha, Big Sean, Taraji P. Henson, Audra McDonald, Brandon Marshall, Michelle Williams, KeKe Palmer, Dr Delvena, Dr Anika, and the millions of ordinary people and celebrity athletes like the beautiful Naomi Osaka and Simone Biles that go through their own struggles and advocate for people that can't speak up for themselves. When someone is mentally drained, and they've conveyed that to friends and family, BELIEVE THEM. People need a break from the stresses of the world. We all need to let our hair down once in a while, but no one should be ridiculed for seeking help or crying out for it. Let's work together to understand these illnesses and break the stigma's surrounding mental health.

LIVE, LAUGH, AND LOVE

www.ingramcontent.com/pod-product-compliance
Lightning Source LLC
Chambersburg PA
CBHW031537210526
45464CB00003B/1050